THE VITAMIN CURE

for Women's Health Problems

HELEN SAUL CASE

ANDREW W. SAUL, PH.D.,
SERIES EDITOR

Basic Health
PUBLICATIONS, INC.

The information contained in this book is based upon the research and personal and professional experiences of the authors. It is not intended as a substitute for consulting with your physician or other healthcare provider. Any attempt to diagnose and treat an illness should be done under the direction of a healthcare professional.

The publisher does not advocate the use of any particular healthcare protocol but believes the information in this book should be available to the public. The publisher and authors are not responsible for any adverse effects or consequences resulting from the use of the suggestions, preparations, or procedures discussed in this book. Should the reader have any questions concerning the appropriateness of any procedures or preparation mentioned, the authors and the publisher strongly suggest consulting a professional healthcare advisor.

Basic Health Publications, Inc.

www.basichealthpub.com

Library of Congress Cataloging-in-Publication Data is available through the Library of Congress.

ISBN-13: 978-1-59120-274-5 (Pbk.)
ISBN-13: 978-1-68162-832-5 (Hardcover)

Editor: Karen Anspach
Typesetting/Book design: Gary A. Rosenberg
Cover design: Mike Stromberg

CONTENTS

ACKNOWLEDGMENTS

Thanks to Ryan, for whose constant love and support I am intensely grateful.

Thanks to both of my parents for their bravery: they dared to raise healthy children with optimal nutrition, megavitamin therapy, and common sense, and by doing so gave me the confidence to doctor myself.

Thanks to Dr. Carolyn Dean, who by her own example through her work and dedication in the field of natural healing, inspired me to enjoy the ride.

Thanks to Robert G. Smith and other editorial review board members of the Orthomolecular Medicine News Service for kind permission to use material from their many news releases.

And thanks again to my father, who always encouraged me to put my words onto paper, and without whom this project would not have been possible.

FOREWORD

When you see your doctor for a health problem, you have an expectation that she or he will help you. However, in a typical seven-minute HMO appointment, you barely have time to get comfortable enough to state your concerns. And forget it if you have three or four symptoms. A doctor will often cut you off after the second problem and tell you to come back for another appointment. But what if all those symptoms are connected and the doctor isn't taking the time to connect the dots? What if poor nutrition is the underlying factor? What if stress is a major concern in your life, causing lots of physical symptoms? If your doctor doesn't understand what's happening in your life, he or she will likely put you on prescription medications instead of counseling you about stress and giving you natural approaches to deal with your symptoms.

What's the most common reaction to drugs? Side effects. Then you are on a prescription drug roller coaster, treating drug side effects with more drugs. Even worse, studies show that most doctors are unable to recognize drug side effects.

Doctors are trained to diagnose disease and treat disease symptoms with drugs. They see symptoms as evidence of disease and they see disease as something that needs to be eradicated with drugs. Preventive medicine to them often means batteries of blood tests and expensive imaging to find early signs of disease. Doctors learn nothing about nutrition, nutrients, or stress management in medical school. In fact, in my training we were warned about the "quackery" of such things as vitamin therapy and herbal remedies. But now I know better. As a physician for over thirty years, I have found the opposite to be true: natural remedies are safe and effective. It is pharmaceuticals that are not.

Luckily for herself, and for us, Helen Saul Case experienced nutritional medicine at work early in her life as she was growing up. But then she confronted allopathic medicine when she left home. She ran up against doctors who don't have time, don't listen, don't know anything about natural remedies, and just reach for the prescription pad. So she decided to look into matters for herself and found that the doctors' drugs were worse than the illnesses. Her reaction was to write this book, *The Vitamin Cure for Women's Health Problems*. She has tapped into a vast body of research and clinical evidence to show that diet, supplements, and natural remedies work, and work well. And you do not just have to take her word for it, for she has provided hundreds of scientific references for substantiation.

Within these pages, Helen writes about her experiences in an engaging manner that speaks directly to you and your needs. Using this book, you can have the best of both worlds. If you wish, you can go to your doctor and use his or her diagnostic tests to find out what's wrong . . . and then use natural alternatives to treat the symptoms.

Do not be misled into thinking that a doctor who gives you seven minutes knows what's best for you. Do your own research and come to your own conclusions. Helen's book offers a way for you to get in touch with your body and take responsibility for your own health. You'll be happy you took her advice.

Carolyn Dean, M.D., N.D.

INTRODUCTION

"When in doubt, try nutrition first."
—ROGER WILLIAMS, PH.D.

I am not a medical doctor, naturopath, nutritionist, dietitian, herbalist, or any kind of physician. My expertise does not lie in the sciences, and I have not had the opportunity to work in a hospital, lab, or the like.

So why am I writing a book about treating illness? And more so, why do I think anyone will *read* it?

I would like to argue that you do not have to be a trained physician to help yourself. If you need to go to the doctor, by all means, go. I certainly have, and their ability to diagnose health problems is valuable, to say the least.

However, after that diagnosis, many patients go home with a slip of paper indicating what prescription to take. Suddenly, it feels like you are on your own . . . because you are. It is not the good doctor helping you every step of the way through your ailment now; you are relying on a drug. And, I daresay, those pills, treatments, ointments, what have you, don't always work, and if they do, so can the side effects. When you experience *this*, all of a sudden modern medicine doesn't seem so brilliant.

As talented and educated as your doctors are, their tool bag is filled with drugs, not vitamins; their solutions are medical solutions;

1

their cures are based on a physician's training. If you seek out natural alternatives, you just won't find them in the tool bag.

You begin to think: If my doctor can't solve this problem, who can? If drugs don't work, what will? How can I get *better*? This is a scary place to be. You are left to fend for yourself.

As I was.

Once I went off to college, out of my parents' nutritional reach, after having not a single dose of antibiotics until I was seventeen, I turned to conventional medicine. It seemed so *easy* to go to the doctor and get a prescription. In fact, it was downright comforting. I thought my parents had really missed the boat.

Soon enough, I found that drugs don't always cure disease. After a while, especially dealing with my own "feminine ailments," not only did drugs not cure what I suffered from, they actually made things worse.

Though I believe some of you will read this book because you are already interested in vitamin cures, I imagine that some of you have turned to this book out of the same frustration I had with drug therapy. Well, perhaps this is to my advantage.

So no, I'm not a doctor, but I am a woman with the will to discover natural vitamin cures because *I needed to*. I have struggled with the fact that women like you and me have few options to turn to when dealing with our own unique health problems. I would like to offer a solution.

This is not a comprehensive textbook to address all women's health issues. It's not even close. This book merely aims to highlight some of the most common health concerns we ladies have and how vitamins and nutrition can help. What you will find in here is a step-by-step drugless approach to a number of the specific illnesses we face. The material is brought to you in a form that is easy to grasp, but by no means "dumbed down." My aim is to discuss these topics with a level of sensitivity and understanding that goes hand in hand with being a woman with a woman's health concerns, a perspective male health book authors just don't have.

When I pick up a book, even if it is easy to navigate and fun to read, I still want lots of scientific support for what the author has to say. Well, I figure you want what I want. I'll be sure to provide lots of research and full citations so you can check and see for yourself that what you have here actually works. What I hope you discover as you read this book is that the information is out there—I've just brought it, in concise, convenient form, into your hands.

I am a writer, a teacher, and a trained administrator. I am sort of an amateur researcher who strives to find solutions to health problems women face, including my own. I happen to have a unique experience growing up in a household where vitamins and nutrition were the answers to our illnesses, and more often, the answer for prevention of illness.

You don't have to take my word for it. The information in this book is the translation of the studies that have already proven vitamins *cure*. I am out to deliver some answers, and I think it is about time that you get to hear them.

CHAPTER 1

NO BOYS ALLOWED

"Without health there is no happiness.
An attention to health, then, should take
the place of every other object."
—THOMAS JEFFERSON

Welcome to our "Ladies Only Health Club." Sorry, guys; there's nothing here for you.

To put it bluntly, unless you have a vagina, you can't possibly know what it is like to deal with one and all the associated health challenges that affect those of us who do.

And really guys, we are going to be talking about chunky yeast infections, head-splitting migraines, bloating, cramps, and funky discharge . . . do you want to hear about these things in detail? Probably not. Just share this book with a girl you know, a girl that is ready to take control of her own health. It is my sincere hope that she will.

Now that the guys have left the room, I welcome the women!

We girls need each other. We need to be able to talk about our health, share our stories, share our advice, our accomplishments, and our angst. We need each other because we *get* each other. We are women, so we identify with women. Men may try to sympathize with our experiences, but they'll never completely understand what we are going through. It's difficult partly because it's so hard to speak to men about problems we have with our bodies; the conversations are uncomfortable, embarrassing, and, well, just so *personal*.

5

I was wading through all these health books written by male authors, and they just can't understand what it's really like being a woman. I wished there was an orthomolecular health book for the kinds of issues I wanted to know about that was written by, well, a woman! Since I couldn't find what I was looking for, I just had to go and write it myself.

There are literally thousands of different health issues out there. Many of these are experienced by both men and women. However, these pages are reserved for the ailments that predominantly affect us ladies because of our unique parts and design. You'll find chapters on the following:

- Menstrual and premenstrual issues such as premenstrual syndrome (PMS), premenstrual dysphoric disorder (PMDD), bloating, stress, cravings, acne, migraines, heavy periods, insomnia, fatigue, breast tenderness, and mood swings

- Bacterial vaginosis

- Yeast infections

- Sex drive concerns

- Urinary tract, bladder, and kidney infections

- Health problems caused by hormonal contraception

- Prevention of female cancers of the breast, ovaries, endometrium, and cervix

- Endometriosis

- Stress, anxiety, and depression

- Menopausal issues such as hot flashes, sweating, vaginal atrophy, vaginal dryness, hair loss, joint discomfort, and urinary incontinence

- Infertility

Keep this book close by. If you are experiencing one of these problems and you feel nervous or scared, take a deep breath and scan through these pages to find natural, drug-free alternatives. You should always go to your doctors with your health concerns, but you don't always have to do what they say. Be informed about your options, and use this book and its references to help you decide what to do.

CHAPTER 2

PMS AND OTHER PERIOD-RELATED PROBLEMS

"I have PMS and a gun . . . now what were you saying?"
—ANONYMOUS (OR JUST CHECK THE POLICE BLOTTER)

The war does not always start out badly. Sometimes battles are won. Other times, our nemesis grabs hold of us, beats us into submission, and refuses to surrender. When the combat is taking place in our own body, we cannot run and we cannot hide. We are forced to fight this uncompromising hormonal torture hoping, in the end, we can sort through the rubble and repair any collateral damage suffered by our job, relationships, and our own sanity.

What is mildly comforting at least is that it is not just "in our head." It is all very biological.

It is also particularly unfair.

I cannot be the only one that has wished, even just for a moment, that perhaps it would have been better to be born a man.

JUST WHAT IS PMS?

Premenstrual syndrome (PMS) is a nice, fancy, medical term to describe a week of hell. And boys just haven't a clue. Perhaps this is a tad unfair as there are many high-quality understanding gentlemen out there. But no matter how wonderful they are, I daresay that sometimes the boys in our life just do not seem to have us or PMS figured out. They accidentally trample upon our delicate moods, causing all sorts of turmoil to transpire. Do they mean to tromp through our proverbial patch of daisies and ceremoniously stomp all over them until they are mashed into an unrecognizable paste? Perhaps not. But unfortunately, even the minor indiscretions of our men (or anyone else for that matter) can expose a most intense female fury when PMS is in town. For some reason, men have been instructed not to diverge from the script they were handed in "How to Handle Her Hormonal Mayhem 101," so they mistakenly remark in response to our slightly erratic behavior: "Honey, are you PMS-ing?"

God help them.

Technically speaking, "PMS is a combination of emotional, physical, psychological, and mood disturbances" that occur after a woman ovulates and before menstruation.[1] I am not sure "disturbances" is a strong enough word. Perhaps "pandemonium" will do; at least it is more polite than swearing.

This premenstrual pandemonium takes no prisoners. If you want to get out of it unscathed (while keeping friends and family protected . . . mostly from you), you will have to arm yourself with nutrition. The goal is to make it through the week in one physical and mental piece. Vitamins can help you do just that.

Symptoms

If I just left blank lines here, I am pretty sure you (or any woman you know) could fill them in without much trouble. But for just for the heck of it, here are some of the symptoms of PMS and its more potent sister PMDD (premenstrual dysphoric disorder): depression, irritability, overreacting, crying, oversensitivity, mood swings, fatigue, bloating, acne, breast tenderness, appetite changes, food cravings, and who knows how many homicides.[2] Apparently there are a lot of ways to spell "miserable."

Risk Factors

Risk factors? How about the obvious one: being a *woman*. And of us gals, 80 percent of us experience at least some level of PMS; 20 to 30 percent suffer intense symptoms, and it is estimated that about 2 to 6 percent of women suffer the more severe symptoms of PMDD.[3] In other words, we're doomed.

To be fair, being a lady is not always so bad. For the first two weeks of our cycle, we feel great. We could take on the world. We feel sexy, confident, and ready for anything.

For the next two weeks, we feel like crap. Headaches, bloating, cramps, moodiness, fatigue, and weight gain occur; we find ourselves flying off the handle at the drop of a hat. Even our closest companions may wish to take cover until the storm clears.

What the heck? Why does this happen?

"Do I Have a Disorder?"

If you do, we all do, and that just doesn't sound quite right. Just because most women experience some level of PMS, it does not mean we are sick. Just because there is a drug for it, does not make it a disease. Just because we experience normal, cyclical changes, does not mean we are defective. Do we need to seek balance and learn to manage our systems so we can live healthy and fulfilling lives? Yes. Do we need to be whacked out on drugs because we have a classifiable "mood disorder"? No. Some of the drugs prescribed for PMS and the more newly branded PMDD are pretty heavy duty. I strongly advise you to seek other ways of treating your PMS symptoms before heading down the pharmaceutical pathway. Since I am pretty sure you read the title of this book before reading this chapter, I can only assume you are heading in the right direction.

DRUGS

"Gimme, gimme, now, now, NOW!" you say?

I hear you. *Really,* I do. When you are PMS-ing, drugs seem very desirable. Anything would that takes the edge off, right?

Our doctors may suggest anything from over-the-counter pain relief to prescription pills for the management of PMS. Diuretics are recommended for bloating and pain killers for cramps and headaches.

Antidepressants are commonly prescribed. Even the birth control pill is used as a menstrual medication rather than a contraceptive. Basically, if you are feeling like a pile of PMS poo, the medical community believes that pumping you full of chemicals will help. I beg to differ.

Let's start with diuretics. I know, I know. Bloating sucks. But is taking the "water pill" *really* the answer? Diuretics help your body get rid of excess salt and water by making your kidneys dump more sodium into your urine. When that excess sodium leaves the body, water is taken with it. There are other more natural ways to rid the body of excess sodium. Not eating too much salt (especially the week before your period, when you have the urge to pound down potato chips) will help and so will other natural methods we will get into later in the chapter.

Nonsteroidal anti-inflammatory drugs (NSAIDs) like ibuprofen might help you battle your headache and other period pains, but side effects should not be ignored. Gastrointestinal irritation is just one of them.[4] This can be pretty uncomfortable. I understand that some of you would rather risk experiencing some "irritation" than suffer through a headache, but what if we could alleviate that headache without just transferring a problem from one part of our body to another? I remember my dad saying to me: "Headache is not due to an aspirin deficiency." Let's address the cause of our pain rather than cover up the symptoms with a drug.

Some women may seek out the birth control pill hoping it can alleviate some of the harsher symptoms of PMS. Acne, cramping; some pills may provide relief.[5] However, for every problem the pill might possibly fix, you may experience just as many other undesirable outcomes. If you want to see just how that is, check out Chapter 6.

Antidepressants are no laughing matter. This is serious mind-altering medication. Selective serotonin reuptake inhibitors (SSRIs) are being increasingly prescribed as a frontline treatment for women suffering from PMS and PMDD.[6] In other words, if you go to your doctor and hand him or her your list of PMS or PMDD mood-related complaints, it is ever more likely that he or she is going to hand you a script for an antidepressant. "Frontline" means that your doctor is

WE'VE GOT A DRUG FOR THAT, TOO. BUT IT'LL COST YA.

"It is easy to get a thousand prescriptions,
but hard to get one single remedy."
—CHINESE PROVERB

I sit here enjoying breakfast, a cup of tea, and my morning television program, and I am inundated with pharmaceutical commercials. I pause to reflect about one of the newer disease names: PMDD, or premenstrual dysphoric disorder. I listen to the symptom checklist and start contemplating. Before long, another disease is presented, along with another pill. Trustworthy voices explain all of the wonderful advantages of taking drugs while charming depictions of nature, enjoyable activities, friends, lovers, and families grace the screen with believable before and after portrayals of hurt transformed into humble success. Some of the commercials are downright heartwarming; they could make a girl get a little teary, especially at this time of the month.

I am awed by the luminous actors, actresses, and doctors (real or otherwise), each playing their pivotal roles creating and selling an image, an idea, and a lifestyle. I also note that, of course, the drug advertisements are broadcast during certain time slots or programs with the obvious expectation that a particular kind of audience will be watching. I see that many of the drugs are intended for older, middle to upper class citizens, the only population that can really afford to be sick.

We are no strangers to advertising. We know the folks behind the commercials are just trying to sell us something. But perhaps we cannot help but wonder how nice it might be if whatever ailment we were struggling with could really be resolved, so simply, so neatly, so efficiently, with one little pill.

Have you ever seen those television ads that simply allude to a name of a drug and do not tell you what it is meant to do? It gets us guessing what mysterious medicine is being marketed. Our curiosity may get the best of us. "What does it do?" we think. If the company does not tell you what it is good for, it appears it also does not have to tell you what is wrong with it either. Eventually, we will see a full-length commercial tells us what this new drug is all about. A thoughtful, calming narrator explains with the utmost sympathy and understanding how a particular health problem can be treated with this wonderful, new, attractively labeled product. And then, when pleasing pictures cross the screen distracting us with their silent stories and smiles, that same soothing voice gently shares a list of potential side effects in such a reassuring manner that it makes us feel as if those things probably wouldn't ever happen to us anyway. We may feel a sense of minimized risk. Our skepticism may wane, and we may find ourselves seeking out a drug that we would not have otherwise thought to pursue. We look for approval from our doctors, and they give it, often with a free sample or two.

Have you ever noticed, as I have, that the side effects of the drugs actually sound *worse* than the conditions they purport to treat? Does it ever make you scratch your head? And yet, there appear to be enough folks out there anxious and hopeful enough to fix one condition that they would risk additional suffering. And this is, of course, assuming that there is a need for treatment in the first place. Are we buying into the idea that we are unwell just because we matched our symptoms with a condition advertised on TV? Critics of the pharmaceutical industry point out that "a lot of money can be made from healthy people who believe they are sick."[8]

Drug ads practically choke out other advertising. They have become an ordinary and expected part of our television shows, our web experience, and the pages of our magazines. Next time you are watching your favorite talk show, game show, or news program, or you are reading your favorite digest or browsing websites—start counting. Literally billions of dollars are spent every year advertising drugs directly to us. And ladies, it works. The most heavily advertised pharmaceuticals see the largest increase in prescriptions and purchases.[9]

Selling directly to the public: it is just brilliant. Create hope in the minds of the consumer and create demand. Create brand recognition, and get people to pay a premium for it. Let's convince the population that they should ask their doctor for the drug they desire. Are the medical professionals holding out on us? We better go tell *them* what we want! It is giving power to the consumer, right? We must be very powerful, because one out of every two people in America is taking prescription meds.[10]

With over a hundred thousand deaths every year due to pharmaceuticals taken as directed,[11] drug companies are pushing products that will have people pushing up daisies. Everywhere in the world, except the United States and New Zealand, this direct-to-consumer advertising is prohibited.[12] We must be lucky, I guess. We are the ones who get to hear about all the latest drugs. We get to ask for them first.

likely to pick an antidepressant *first*. Being overwhelmingly moody is not any fun, and for women seeking cures, an antidepressant might not look so bad. Consider, though, as with any drug, antidepressants come with their own list of issues, some perhaps just as troublesome as the symptoms being treated: gastrointestinal problems, drowsiness, nausea, loss of appetite, anxiety, insomnia, headaches, and—this one is really not nice—reduced sex drive. Check out the list of side effects for some of the most commonly prescribed SSRIs like Zoloft, Prozac (also called Sarafem, renamed for its application in PMDD), and Paxil. They might help with your mood, but they do not necessarily help your bodily symptoms and can rather *cause* you to suffer physical side effects.[7]

And what if you are pregnant or want to be? None of these medical treatment options sound good if there is going to be a baby involved. We need to look to nutritional approaches for managing PMS if we really want to feel better. To improve your sense of well-being and combat PMS effectively without drugs, a good diet and exercise are needed, and so are vitamins.

WHAT TO STOP DOING

Nobody really likes to be told what they cannot do, particularly when they are not in the mood to receive advice, but if you find yourself feeling especially charitable at the moment, take a minute and read through what you need to stop doing in order to start feeling better.

Just not eating right can intensify PMS symptoms.[13] Women who experience severe PMS tend to ingest sodium, caffeine, and refined carbohydrates.[14] So, for starters, cut out some sweets and white flour. Data suggest that there is a link between sugar intake and the prevalence and severity of PMS.[15] We know we should be avoiding refined sugar (the kind in candy, not the kind in fruit) and refined carbohydrates (such as those in white flour instead of good-for-you whole grains and other complex carbs). We are not talking about elimination, at least not yet, just *reduction* of the bad stuff. Have a piece or two of dark chocolate instead of the entire candy bar. And put. The chips. Down. Avoiding salt before your menstrual period may help reduce bloating.[16] Increased sodium intake equals water retention and weight gain. Lastly, don't wait to eat. Eating several small meals a day will help keep your blood-sugar in check.

Reduce your caffeine intake. One study found that caffeine is strongly related to severe PMS symptoms: the more caffeine you take in, the more likely it is that you will be suffering.[17] I know, it is easy to get hooked on your favorite coffee and teas; they taste and smell so good! It becomes a social ritual, a comfort, to hold a warm cup and sip a hot beverage. No doubt, we know how stimulating caffeine can be. Don't feel too bad about submitting to its allure. You are not alone. It is estimated that 80 percent of the world takes in caffeine every single day.[18] We need to remember that caffeine is a drug, one we can become dependent on[19] and one we can suffer withdrawal symptoms from when we cease to use it, even if we ingest a low or moderate amount.[20] Plus, caffeinated beverages may displace other, healthier drinks. If you are having trouble sleeping at night, as some folks do when they drink caffeine,[21] or you get headaches when you do not get your daily dose, these may be signs that you need to eliminate it from your diet. If you are already an anxious person, adding a stimulant to your system may not be the best idea either. Cut back on the caffeine; see if it is related to your PMS symptoms.

Reduce your alcohol intake. All that drinking may make you feel good in the moment, but it is more harmful to your mood in the long run. Alcohol affects both your intake and absorption of B vitamins, nutrients that are essential for keeping you in good spirits. As discussed by Abram Hoffer, M.D., Ph.D., and Andrew W. Saul, Ph.D., in *The Vitamin Cure for Alcoholism,* "Thiamine (B_1) is needed for carbohydrate metabolism. Extra carbohydrates, including alcohol, require extra thiamine. Because alcohol is filling, it displaces more nourishing foods in the diet, causing malnutrition and specifically causing thiamine deficiency. So, the heavy drinker is much less likely to get even the usual dietary amount of thiamine at a time when he or she needs much more. Still worse, alcohol causes poor absorption and poor utilization of what B vitamins there are."[22] Help yourself out by cutting back on the booze.

Quit smoking. Nuff said. There are about a million reasons to quit but here are a few more. You are more at risk for having menstrual cramps if you smoke,[23] and it has been shown that just environmental exposure to cigarette smoke can increase your risk of getting menstrual cramps.[24] This means you are at risk even if you are not the one puffing away. Smoking may be making your period much more unbearable. Women who smoke report having the worst menstrual issues.[25] In fact, women who smoke are *two times* more likely to develop PMS than never-smokers.[26] Starting young also increases your chances of developing moderate to severe PMS.[27] Are you lighting that ciggie to feel better? Well, put it out sister, because it is not helping.

If you are already trying to quit, that's awesome. Bolster your effort with vitamins A, B, C, D, and E and a good multi.

SALT AND SUGAR, SUGAR AND SALT

Like clockwork, Audrey would take a ride on the salt-sugar roller-coaster the week before her period. As soon as the salt craving was satisfied, her sugar craving would kick in, and then she was back to wanting salt. Willpower is a tough thing to wrangle up when all you really want to do is wolf down package of Bridge Mix. Must we deny ourselves joy? No, but we should limit how much "joy" we eat!

Okay, so none of these suggestions are going to make you happy right now per se, but if you can harness the willpower to say *no*, do so. Then, when PMS time rolls around, you'll have set yourself up to feel well.

ARMED AND READY: WHAT TO START DOING TO KICK SOME PM-ASS

It is time to start feeling better for three or more months out of every year. Let's break it down. Here is a brief overview of what you need to do to help alleviate your PMS symptoms.

Ceasing the Stress

PMS symptoms are emotional and physical, and you have to address both in order to feel better, starting with getting up out of your chair. Premenstrual boot camp requires exercise. You *need* to get out and move around. It is amazing how much better you will feel if you just make yourself do it. Exercise boosts your mood by increasing your serotonin levels,[28] and it also helps you to reduce stress. Since PMS is stress-related, you will experience fewer PMS symptoms if you get up and exercise.[29] We all know that exercise can help burn away those pesky pounds. Being really overweight is also strongly associated with PMS.[30] Even if you are feeling tired and lethargic, put in the effort to be active anyway. You will be surprised how much more energy you have (and how much better you feel mentally) afterwards. It is something about doing the right thing, knowing it is the right thing, and being proud for getting it done. Take a walk, go for a bike ride, do some gardening, move the couch and get out that yoga mat. Improve your mood, get a better night's sleep, and hey—your figure will benefit too!

Exercise is just one of the many lifestyle changes that can lessen stress. A warm bath, spending some time outdoors, writing out your thoughts, talking with a good friend, getting a massage, aromatherapy, listening to music, meditation, reading, getting enough sleep, watching something on TV or the Internet that gets you laughing are all effective stress reducers.

Vitamins can help, too. Vitamin C (ascorbic acid) can actually help you withstand stress.[31] When the body is under any kind of strain, be it mental, physical, or chemical, (hello! PMS!?) our need for vitamin C increases.[32] Unlike most animals on earth that can just create more vitamin C under stressful conditions, we cannot.[33] So, we should supplement when we stress out. Start by taking 2,000

VITAMIN D₃

It is no surprise that you feel better after being in the sun for a little while; vitamin D can enhance your mood and just make you feel better. Women with premenstrual syndrome happen to have lower levels of vitamin D;[36] getting more in your diet is associated with a lower prevalence of PMS.[37] According to Dr. Michael Holick, about one billion people worldwide are deficient in D. He recommends taking a dose of 1,000 international units (IU) a day, or get some sunlight: about five to ten minutes a day three times a week.[38] In one large study, women who take more vitamin D (around 700 IU per day) had a reduced risk for PMS.[39] Getting a sufficient amount of Vitamin D not only helps PMS symptoms but is also associated with a reduced risk for cancer, diabetes, and multiple sclerosis.[40] Let's hear it for D!

milligrams (mg) of vitamin C three times a day a day with meals; you can adjust your intake higher or lower based on how you feel. If you are more comfortable starting with a smaller dose, you could take 500–1,000 mg at each meal, and gradually work up to 2,000 mg or more. Keep in mind that vitamin C is not dangerous even in very large quantities.[34]

B vitamins, especially niacin (B_3) and pyridoxine (B_6), and zinc should also be part of your stress-reduction nutrient cocktail.[35] They also happen to be helpful for other symptoms of PMS.

Eat Well

Instead of eating sugar-laden and salt-laden foods, stick to a low animal fat, high-fiber diet. It has been suggested that more research is needed to determine the benefits of a low-fat, high-fiber diet to assess whether or not it works for PMS.[41] Come now, is there really not enough research out there to demonstrate why healthy eating is a good idea? Well, there is some. One study found that a low-fat vegetarian diet helped women lose weight, lessen the discomfort and duration of menstrual cramps, and reduce the time spent with PMS symptoms.[42] It's not exactly a wild idea to suggest that eating right might make you feel better. In fact, it just might work!

Maybe we eat junk foods because we ourselves feel like garbage. Maybe when we feel bad and we also do not eat right, we set ourselves up to feel worse. I have wanted to double up and vomit out a bag of red-painted, plastic-textured candy twists before (ah, youth), but I have never felt that way after having a salad with my favorite dressing. Eat several small meals a day. Focus on reducing bad fats, salt, and refined sugar, and increase your fiber intake.

Curtail Your Cramps

Sometimes your cramps may be minor and just feel like someone has a gentle fistful of your bowels; other times, your cramps might be so bad you cannot even move—we are talking stop-you-dead-in-your-tracks-take-a-day-off-of-work cramps. Some of you are no strangers to the feeling that makes you want to double over and huddle in a little ball all afternoon because your insides have been tied in a knot. Cramps can be accompanied by headache, nausea, vomiting, and an intense desire to remove the lower half of your body. Unfortunately, you can get abdominal cramps during PMS and while menstruating. We can also cramp up at other times and in other places, too. Whether they radiate from our abdomen, legs, or another place, from mildly obnoxious to downright crippling, cramps can really ruin your day. Wouldn't it be nice if you could get rid of cramps *before* they start? Instead of just treating them, let's be done with them all together.

Standard medical procedure for your basic menstrual cramp (dysmenorrhoea) is to recommend a conventional anti-inflammatory pain reliever, but they will not work for as many as one in five of us.[43] For women with severe menstrual cramps, doctors may suggest oral contraceptives (OCs), even to adolescent girls;[44] however, there is little evidence showing that OCs help pain from dysmenorrhoea.[45] Even if you are lucky and experience some relief from your cramps while on the pill, OCs come with their own laundry list of side effects. There are natural alternatives that can work without the side effects of taking drugs.

If you have been suffering from cramps, the following suggestions are probably not new to you, but if you have not tried them, do so. Exercise can really help your mood and help alleviate stress. Since stress can affect the severity of your cramps, it makes sense to give it a try.[46] I know; if you cannot even move, that is not much of a suggestion, but if you can, you should! Walk the dog, clean the garage, or chase the kids around the yard. Be sure you are drinking enough water, too. Some women may find relief with massage therapy and yoga, other stress-reducing activities. A warm bath or a heating pad may relax tense muscles. Applying heat may be as good if not better than taking ibuprofen or acetaminophen for menstrual pain.[47] Get enough sleep, too. You might want to try acupuncture.[48] Even orgasms can help ease the pain.[49] That is a good one to try first.

Now here is what you may not have tried for cramps: magnesium. Several studies have shown that magnesium may help curtail cramps.[50] Ladies who have tried it know: magnesium is extremely effective for getting rid of that pain in the gut! Nuts, soybeans, beans, spinach and other green leafy veggies all contain a measure of magnesium, but we ladies still do not get even the recommended amount of over 300 mg per day.[51] To kick cramps to the curb, you are going to need more than that. Start taking 300 mg of magnesium *twice* a day, every day.[52] This is in addition to the magnesium you may already be getting from your food. You can also take a bath. Patented in 1999, therapeutic bath salts containing magnesium sulfate were indicated for the relaxation of muscles and reduction of muscle spasms.[53] Grandma knew well before 1999 that a super-relaxing way to get a megadose of magnesium is by taking a bath with Epsom salts (also known as magnesium sulfate) to soothe aches and pains. There's nothing quite like a warm soak to calm tense, tight muscles. It becomes easier to sleep at night, as well as face your busy days.

Supplement your magnesium intake with an equal amount of additional calcium, at least 600 mg per day.[54] One study involving hundreds of women showed that getting 1,200 mg per day of calcium significantly helped PMS pain symptoms.[55]

Another natural option is to take vitamin E. Women taking 200 IU of vitamin E twice a day beginning two days before the expected start date of menstruation and then continuing through the first three days of their period, experienced less pain from menstrual cramps.[56]

CHARLEY HORSES

Have you ever woken up in the middle of the night because you get a cramp in your leg that is so bad you swear someone just took a baseball bat to it? There is nothing quite like being awakened from a deep, peaceful rest, with tight, twisting pain in your calf. And it does not end there. Your leg might be sore for days to come. I used to get "charley horses" as my mom called them, and they feel just *awful*. The good news is, once I started taking more magnesium, I never had one again.

Thiamine (B_1) helped hundreds of women completely eliminate dysmenorrhoea when they took 100 mg per day.[57] Supplementation with iron and niacin (B_3) may also help out menstrual cramps[58] as can the omega-3 fatty acids taken alone[59] or in conjunction with B_{12}.[60] A daily intake of 200 mg of B_6 has also been shown to be helpful.[61] You may be able to reduce or eliminate your need for drugs by using these safe and natural nutrient-based alternatives. You may even just rid yourself of cramps, period. That sounds pretty good to me.

Halt Those Headaches

I am not sure what makes life stop faster than a bad headache. Even the simplest of tasks . . . walking . . . talking . . . all become a trial. You muddle through your workday, periodically downing pain pills, just to come home and crash, unable to do anything for the rest of the evening. Headaches can be a bit bothersome to downright debilitating. Some may just be minor pains in the neck; others are massive migraines that move in for days and limit all activity. Sometimes they may show up randomly; sometimes we know exactly what days we are going to get them. Women are far more likely to get a migraine headache than men, and millions of us will, even as often as one or more a month.[62] We will cost the health care system lots of money; we will cost our employers billions from lost work days.[63] Teaming up with our period, menstrual migraines can really take the fun out of life.

It may be hard to rid yourself of a hormonal headache, but there is a lot you can do to make them more bearable. Magnesium and migraines are linked, so there is another really good reason to be taking it every day. In one study, women taking 360 mg per day of magnesium (the current United States Recommended Dietary Allowance (RDA) for women ages fourteen to eighteen) experienced some relief from menstrual migraines and PMS complaints.[64] Women in this study who took magnesium also had a headache for a *fewer number of days*.[65] I don't know about you, but I would be thrilled to knock a day or two off of a splitting headache. Data suggest that magnesium deficiency may cause you to have a lower threshold for migraines.[66] We can interpret this in a positive way: if we are getting enough magnesium, we will not be so sensitive to headache triggers. Other nutrients are important too. Calcium, vitamin D, chromium, omega-3 fatty acids, vitamin C and B vitamins, like B_2 and B_3,[67] may all play a role in helping halt your headache.[68]

Other natural helpers you may want to try include a visit to your chiropractor or acupuncturist. Make sure you are drinking enough water to rule out that your headache is due to dehydration. Down a glass or two of water and see how you feel in twenty minutes. If you suffer from migraines, you know there are certain "triggers" that can set you off, such as lack of food or sleep, stress, anxiety, changes in the weather, chocolate, alcohol, monosodium glutamate (MSG), nitrates, and so on, so do your best to avoid them. Stress, for example, is a biggie. Whatever you can do to reduce stress may help you stop the migraine before it gets worse, or may shorten its duration. A shower, a bath, fresh air and sunlight, exercise, meditation, a nap, a good night's sleep, massage, a hot or cold compress: all may help.

Some folks who use homeopathic remedies experience relief from migraine.[69] Ready-to-use migraine relief tablets are available on the market. They typically contain certain botanical and mineral ingredients like belladonna, Cimicfuga racemosa, Gelsemium, Natrum muriaticum, Iris versicolor, Bryonia, Sanguinaria, and Silicea. The argument against homeopathic remedies is, "Well, it is just a placebo effect." Okay, but the placebo effect occurs with conventional medication, too, and some argue it is just about as prevalent as it is in homeopathy.[70] Think about it: some people are *feeling better,* and without the potential risks of using prescription drugs. Perhaps migraine is partly a state of mind—pun intended. My thought is, if homeopathic remedies can work for some people, they may work for you too. Something that is quite safe (a lot safer that conventional meds),[71] inexpensive, and does not cause side effects—sounds like something worth trying.

For more about vitamins cures for these tough headaches, I recommend you check out *The Vitamin Cure for Migraines: How to Prevent and Treat Migraine Headaches Using Nutrition and Vitamin Supplementation* by Steve Hickey, Ph.D.

Fight Fatigue

Ugh. It is that feeling you get when you just do not have the energy for *anything*. (I am proud of you for picking up this book!) There is much you can do to battle fatigue. If you know you are getting enough rest, it is time to start looking at nutrition for the cause behind the symptom.

Analyze your sugar and caffeine intake. You may want to cut back on your consumption if you find yourself crashing after the stimulating effects wear off. Perhaps you think I must be nuts to even suggest limiting caffeine when you already feel so tired and you swear it's the only thing keeping you conscious. I know it sounds a tad crazy. Stick with me and keep reading.

Investigate your iron intake. Ladies, we are losing iron every month. When we have our period, we lose blood (about three pints a year) and iron goes with it. It is not uncommon to be deficient in iron, especially if you are born a girl.[72] The National Heart, Lung, and Blood Institute, a division of the National Institutes of Health and U.S. Department of Health and Human Services, estimates that one in five women suffer from iron-deficiency anemia,[73] the most common symptom of which is fatigue.[74] Being low on iron can also make it harder to process thoughts, learn, remember, and pay attention.[75] Yes, you can get enough iron from your diet, but so many of us obviously are not. Help fight fatigue with iron supplements.[76] Find an iron supplement in the form of ferrous fumarate, ferrous gluconate, or as carbonyl iron. Avoid ferrous sulfate; it will probably make you feel sick.

> If you are worried about getting too much iron, take a moment to read the excerpt on the next page by Andrew W. Saul, Ph.D., from his book, *Doctor Yourself: Natural Healing that Works,* 2012 revised edition.

Another vitamin you will want to start taking is C. For one, vitamin C helps your body absorb iron. In addition, folks with low intakes of vitamin C reported twice as many symptoms of fatigue compared to those who took more.[77]

Iron Overload, or Meat Overload?

Too much blood iron has been associated with an increase in heart disease.[1] On the other hand, a study published in the *New England Journal of Medicine*[2] by the National Center for Health Statistics and Centers for Disease Control reported that "high transferrin saturation levels are not associated with an increased risk of cardiovascular heart disease or myocardial infarction. On the contrary, it was found that there is an inverse association of iron stores with overall mortality and with mortality from cardiovascular disease."[3]

In other words, high iron does not cause cardiovascular disease, but low iron actually might. Health is somewhere in the middle.

Twenty years ago, always a shameless promoter of vegetarianism, I taught my clinical nutrition students that there were two types of dietary iron: heme, and non-heme. That basically means "blood," and "non-blood." Heme iron is from meat.

Your body can soak up and accumulate excessive heme iron even if it already has plenty of iron on hand.

But the really good news is that your body has an automatic shut-off system to limit its absorption of non-heme, or vegetarian, iron. Yes, this includes practically all iron supplements on Earth (and those that may someday be made from meteors as well).

Do I think you should take an iron supplement, or a multiple vitamin containing iron? If you are a child, yes. Iron deficiency remains a major public health problem for kids, because they are making lots of blood as they grow. If you are a reproductive aged female, yes again. Women lose about a half a cup of blood in every menstrual cycle. That's like giving a unit of blood three times a year, ladies.

But this is no reason to stuff women and children with the muscles of dead animals. A simple, cheap multivitamin with iron will do the trick and save a cow. Vegetarianism (or in my personal opinion, what I call "near-vegetarianism") has always been a good idea. Now it is better than ever.

For men, iron supplementation is generally unnecessary. For heme-heavy "meat and potatoes men," it is positively a bad idea. Guys, if you give blood a lot, persistently do excessively heavy exercise, or lose blood from injury, take any average-dose iron supplement for a while.

Caution: These above comments, while valid for the great majority of people, do not apply to persons with hereditary hemochromatosis, which is a severe iron-buildup problem. Next time you have your blood checked, you can bring this up with your doctor of choice.

References

1. Ascherio, A., W. C. Willett, E. B. Rimm, et al. "Dietary Iron Intake and Risk of Coronary Heart Disease among Men." *Circulation* 89 (1994):969–974.

2. Sempos, C. T., A. C. Looker, R. F. Gillum, et al. "Body Iron Stores and the Risk of Coronary Heart Disease." *N Eng J Med* 330 (1994): 1119–1124.

3. Germano, C. "Iron Status and Cardiovascular Heart Disease: New Data! More Confusion!" http://www.drpasswater.com/nutrition_library/iron_heart.html. (accessed November 2011).

B vitamins can help battle fatigue, so here is yet another reason to grab that B-complex vitamin.[78]

You may also feel overtired and lethargic because you need more magnesium. Some chronic fatigue patients were found to have lower levels of magnesium in their blood. Magnesium treatment improved their energy, mood, and pain symptoms.[79]

Zinc, selenium, and omega fatty acids (omega-3 and omega-6) are other nutrients worth obtaining to help fight off fatigue.[80]

If you are suffering from chronic fatigue, I would recommend that you read Dr. Jonathan Prousky's book *The Vitamin Cure for Chronic Fatigue Syndrome.*

OMEGA-3 AND OMEGA-6: BALANCE IS IMPORTANT

Omega-6 fatty acids are present in refined vegetable oils common to many snack foods, cookies, and other processed foods. Omega-3 fatty acids are not as easy to obtain in the typical American diet. They are found in fish such as salmon, mackerel, herring, tuna, scallops, sardines, and in vegetarian sources like kidney beans, pinto beans, flaxseeds, winter squash, spinach, broccoli, walnuts, and olive oil. Due to the relatively small number of food sources for omega-3, it is likely that your diet mirrors that of most Americans: it has more omega-6 fatty acids and not enough omega-3. Consider supplementation with omega-3 to better complement the omega-6 you already ingest.

IRON AND FATIGUE: MOM KNOWS BEST

I used to watch my mom conk out on the couch in the middle of a conversation. It started to bug me, especially when I had all sorts of things I wanted her to patiently listen to, so one day I just asked her if she was getting enough iron. She realized that she indeed was not getting enough, and started taking iron supplements.

Just this past year, I was complaining about being fatigued. I had the energy to do just about nothing and I could only blame so much on the fact that I taught eighth grade. Teaching certainly drains energy, but the kind of tiredness I was experiencing was even more profound. I was getting enough sleep, I was exercising, and I was eating right. One day while I was chatting on the phone with my mom, she burst out, "Well are YOU taking enough iron?" By golly, I wasn't. Not a big eater of meat or fortified cereals, I could not figure out where iron would enter my diet in sufficient amounts. I immediately remedied the situation by taking 27 mg of iron fumarate and the fatigue vanished *that day*. I now take iron every day, and it has not come back.

Ban Bloating

Bloating, otherwise known as "Damn, these pants used to fit" is another lovely symptom that is like a kick in the ass when you are down and already not feeling all that sexy. According to Dr. Carolyn Dean, "Fluid retention is a big part of PMS, so it's a good idea to avoid foods that contain salt and sugar and therefore exacerbate water retention. That means that chips, sugar, desserts, alcohol, tea, coffee, soft drinks, and processed foods are out . . . . Try to eat an optimum diet of whole grains, nuts, seeds, vegetables, legumes, fish, and chicken."[81] Like it or not, ladies, that is what you will have to do if you want to wear *those* jeans. Dr. Dean also recommends that you take B_6 to the tune of 100–300 mg per day in divided doses, along with a daily multivitamin (mostly for the B vitamin content to balance the additional B_6 you're taking) to decrease fluid buildup.[82] Additionally, 200 mg of magnesium per day (that is not even the RDA for women age nine to ninety-nine) was shown to help reduce weight gain, bloating, and swelling of hands and legs.[83] Calcium, in doses of 1,000–1,200 mg per day, significantly alleviated water retention and pain in women with PMS.[84] You need to get enough potassium, too, which is one more reason to eat tons of fruits and veggies. Prunes and bananas, for example, pack quite a potassium punch.

Curb Your Cravings

Cravings. Are these bad? Is there anything better than *wanting* chocolate, actually *locating* chocolate, and *eating* chocolate? Nothing is quite as satisfying as a craving that has been fulfilled until . . . after it is fulfilled. Did you really want the chocolate bar? Yes! But did you really want to *eat it,* now that you already have? We know we should eat right and cut back our intake of salt and sugar, but it is a battle of wills: mind versus body. Sometimes we lose our ability to say "no" because, frankly, if we are PMS-ing, we want to eat something that makes us feel better.

Speaking of which, there might be more to that chocolate hankering of yours. Chocolate happens to be most frequently craved food

TIRED? CRAVING SUGAR? HEADACHE?

If you are fatigued, achy, anxious, depressed, irritable, headachy, crave sugar, and/or feel spaced-out, do not rule out the possibility that yeast (*candida-albicans*) is to blame. This is especially true for those of you who have taken antibiotics or hormonal birth control. Other yeast-related symptoms include recurrent urinary tract infections (UTIs), recurrent yeast infections, painful sex, loss of interest in sex, burning vulva, endometriosis, infertility, cystitis, and—you may have guessed it—PMS. Check out the chapter on yeast infections and *The Yeast Connection and Women's Health* by Dr. William Crook and Dr. Carolyn Dean.

around this neck of the woods, and its magnesium content and other mood-altering properties may be especially why women crave it more than men.[85] Chocolate is high in magnesium,[86] an essential mineral that alleviates so many PMS symptoms. Could there be a link here? Well, if we are craving magnesium, why aren't we craving halibut or mixed nuts?[87] There must be something about chocolate, and my guess is we want it because it usually comes attached to sugar and fat. You cannot ignore the fact that it has a great texture and smells good, too. To help curb those chocolate cravings, be sure to get magnesium through other healthier foods and through supplements. Do not feel you have to deny yourself all things tasty; just cut back on the things you know are not as healthy. You do not want too much of one food displacing another you should be eating.

In addition to keeping *what* you eat in check, consider *how* you eat, too. Eating small, frequent meals will help balance your blood sugar so you won't lose your temper and break into the snack machine for a fix. The mineral chromium may help out with your carbohydrate cravings and increased appetite.[88] Take 200–400 mcg (that's micrograms) of chromium every day, especially if you have any hint of hypoglycemia.[89] This is all the more important because 90 percent of us are eating chromium deficient diets.[90] Find a chromium

CALCIUM

If you have ever stuffed yourself on pickles and cheese and called it dinner, or started to eat mustard right out of the jar, you may want to investigate your calcium intake. I am not ashamed to admit that many a meal has started with such snacking on my part. Vinegar, a weak acid, helps dissolve calcium, so that pickle or mustard craving might be your body's way of telling you that calcium supplements should also be on the menu. Taking more calcium (for example, carbonate or citrate) means less PMS. A large study found that women who get about 1,280 mg per day of calcium reduced their risk for PMS when compared with women who were only getting about 530 mg per day.[93] Another study showed that a 1,000 mg calcium supplement taken every day significantly reduced PMS symptoms.[94] Hundreds of women in yet another study showed that 1,200 mg of calcium a day significantly reduced PMS symptoms, with a big effect on cravings for sweets or salt,[95] and even taking twice that much is very safe.[96] Calcium has also been shown to significantly help reduce water retention and pain during PMS.[97]

The government thinks we should be getting about 1,000–1,300 mg per day of calcium in our diets.[98] Well, are we? Surprise, surprise; no, we aren't. Not even with all that extra cheese we put on our mustard. Most of us ladies at risk for PMS are not getting enough calcium. In fact, according to stats from The National Health and Nutrition Examination Survey 1999–2000, women aged twelve to sixty are only getting somewhere between 660 and 797 mg per day.[99] This is an easy one to fix. Calcium is cheap, effective, and safe, even for pregnant gals. Excessively high levels of calcium in the blood can cause hypercalcemia, but this is rarely caused by dietary calcium or supplements.[100] Divide your doses, and take it every day with magnesium (they need each other). You may find your pickle 'n' cheese grocery bill is dramatically reduced.

complex with niacin (to enhance absorption) or take chromium picolinate. If you are looking for the best food source of chromium, eat Brewer's or "nutritional" yeast. To help curb cravings and help control blood sugar levels, chromium is safe and worth trying.

Another helpful supplement is vitamin E. Taking 400 IU of vitamin E a day was shown to significantly improve cravings during PMS.[91] Calcium supplementation (1,200 mg per day) may also be very helpful for reducing PMS-related food cravings.[92]

Baby Your Breasts

Our boobs. Sigh. These poor puppies put up with so much. From unrelenting scrutiny and societal judgment, to being constricted with oppressive contraptions, to groping from babies and the stud muffin you married . . . they truly have had no rest. And now, as if justified, they hurt. "Don't even think of touching us," they say. "We've had enough." And they have. So what can we do to take care of the girls when they need us the most? Yes, there are vitamins for them too! In one study, taking 200 mg per day of magnesium helped reduce breast tenderness and provided other PMS relief as well.[101] Vitamin E may also help reduce PMS breast symptoms.[102] Lifestyle changes can help, too. Some women report relief from breast pain when they cut back their caffeine intake.[103] The omega-6 fatty acids found in evening primrose oil may help women with tender breasts;[104] although results have been mixed, it may be worth giving it a try. Be sure to keep up with regular self-check breast exams. Anything unusual, like lumps or discharge, should be evaluated by your doc. For general breast health, eating a high-fiber, low animal fat diet (that'll help you stay regular, too), avoiding caffeine, and losing excess weight are all worthy considerations.

Alleviate Acne

Acne is icky and all too familiar to us during our special womanly weeks. If I had the solution for acne in a bottle, I would probably be a millionaire, and certainly there are folks out there working on exactly that. We know about keeping our face clean and steering away from chemicals and products that clog our pores. But even on a face that is as sterile as a laboratory clean room, somehow zits still seem to form. It is no surprise that so many of us turn to prescriptions for help.

We can blame female hormones at least in part for our acne-related woes. Women are more likely to get acne later in life (thirties and beyond) than guys are.

Do you ever notice that when your diet is poor, so is your complexion? Think about the kinds of foods we are drawn to during PMS. Perhaps acne is purely a result of our hormones or perhaps there is a dietary connection. One function of your skin is to get rid of wastes. If you are eating lots of bad-for-you food, it makes sense that your skin may have to contend with your choices. It never hurts to drink lots of water and eat right, so try a nutrient-packed diet. Eating low-sugar, high-fiber meals, drinking lots of fresh vegetable juices, and taking vitamins will help keep your face looking clear. Exercise, too, may help sweat out the junk instead of having it show up in bumps on your face.

Vitamins can help. Supplementing your diet with vitamins B_3 and B_6 (try a B-complex), vitamin C, and the mineral zinc, while avoiding foods that contain sugar, will help clear mild to severe acne in most people.[105] Magnesium and vitamin E may help, too. All of those nutrients just happen to be helpful for other symptoms of PMS. Once one PMS problem starts to go away with nutritional therapy, watch others, like acne, fade with it. To get started with vitamin supplementation, check out the section "The Right Pills for PMS."

Be careful when using oral contraceptives that promise relief from acne. All hormonal contraceptives come with the risk of a number of side effects that are not so pleasant. Okay, so your face may clear up, but is it really worth it? Perhaps you can try something else far less drastic than medication first.

Manage Your Mood

It can be maddening trying to compromise with your head. Logically, you know you should not be flying off the handle. You can almost step back and *watch* yourself lose it. It appears to make no difference, though. That brief moment of consciousness where you acknowledge you are indeed PMS-ing does not seem to help you to manage the moment any better.

"I am PMS-ing. I should stop." Yeah right.

My best friend once said that telling someone to take vitamins when they are irritable is like being told to "take your *bad mood* pill because you're in a *bad mood*!"

She's right. Very few of us in a bad mood want to be told so, but if we can learn to know the difference between just being a little upset and being irrationally over-the-top ticked, we can start to intervene with vitamins. Sure, it is okay to be upset once in a while. It is not okay to lose it because PMS is driving you mad, especially when there is something you can do about it.

From depression to elation, apprehension to tranquility, mood swings might be one of the most unbearable PMS symptoms for you and those who know you. Other symptoms of PMS are pretty private; you could say nothing and no one would really know that you are bloated, cramping, tired, and suffering from a headache. Even if you did make an announcement, many folks would think you are just having a rough day. But add mood swings into the mix and every-one becomes pretty sure that you must be PMS-ing. Needless to say, hopefully they keep this observation to themselves.

Magnesium, in doses of 200–1,080 mg per day, has been shown to help women with PMS mood changes, anxiety, irritability, and nervous tension.[106] One study showed that 400 IU of vitamin E a day can significantly improve PMS moods.[107] Vitamin B_6 in doses of 50–200 mg per day may also help with PMS mood symptoms.[108] In general, the B vitamins are going to be a helpful bunch. Take a B-complex along with that extra B_6 and even extra B_3 (in the form of niacinamide, as it may be more effective for anxiety than other forms of niacin)[109] for those trying moments. Vitamin D, the kind your body makes from sunlight, has been shown to help folks be less depressed.[110] Vitamin D not only helps the "winter blues", but data suggest that it may also help PMS symptoms.[111] Calcium

B$_6$ TO THE RESCUE!

People do not necessarily mean to piss us off while we are PMS-ing; it just seems to happen all that much easier. Thank goodness for B$_6$.

Touchy?

Tense?

Troubled?

Tired?

Temperamental?

How many of those did you just check off? If you are suffering from symptoms like these, you might need B$_6$, also called pyridoxine. Women with premenstrual anxiety, irritability, and nervous tension have elevated levels of estrogen and low progesterone.[113] B$_6$ reduces blood estrogen levels, increases progesterone, and improves PMS symptoms.[114] Working with folate, B$_{12}$, and tryptophan in order to make serotonin, B$_6$ is an essential vitamin that you need to help you feel better. Give your body the proper materials so it can manufacture the product you need.

If you *really* pay attention to what you are eating, it is possible to get the low 1.3–2.0 mg per day indicated by the RDA through our consumption of such foods as whole grains, chicken, bananas, nuts, potatoes, and spinach. But if you want to battle PMS, there is plenty of evidence that indicates 50–200 mg of B$_6$ a day is safe and effective.[115] Wait a minute—that is 25 to 100 times the RDA. Is taking all that extra B$_6$ okay? Yes. It is a whole lot safer than having millions of angry women on the loose for one week out of every month. All kidding aside, it also happens to be safer than the prescription drugs you might consider taking. When you are really feeling volatile, adding 50–200 mg of extra B$_6$ to your diet is very unlikely to cause any side effects, especially when taken in conjunction with a B-complex.[116] Problems experienced from overdoses do occur, but they are rare and generally only happen when large amounts (2,000–6,000 mg) are taken every day for an extended period of time. These neurological side effects are temporary and go away once dosages are reduced.[117] Dr. Alan Gaby points out that "[P]yridoxine neurotoxicity has been known to the medical profession for 20 years, and because vitamin B_6 is being taken by millions of people, it is reasonable to assume that neurotoxicity at doses below 200 mg per day would have been reported by now, if it does occur at those doses. The fact that no such reports have appeared strongly suggests that vitamin B_6 does not damage the nervous system when taken at doses below 200 mg per day."[118] The benefits of B_6 substantially outweigh the risks.

Frankly, I am not in the mood to eat thirty cans of garbanzo beans in order to score a therapeutic 200 mg dose of B_6. Nothing against chickpeas, I just do not have the time or the energy to do all that chewing. In my case, it is far more likely the cans would become projectiles aimed at unsuspecting bystanders rather than be eaten by me in search of a happier self. Supplements sure are handy for the girl on the go.

Don't forget the other Bs. Working together, the B vitamins do a great job of settling our sour moods. For PMS symptoms, it is recommended that you take a B-complex that contains 50 mg each of B_1, B_2, B_3 and B_6.[119] The other Bs—B_{12}, biotin (B_7), pantothenic acid (B_5), and folic acid (B_9)—are important too, and will usually come in doses that complement the other concentrations of B vitamins in your supplement.

supplementation (1,200 mg per day) along with alleviating bloating and pain, has also been shown to help relieve mood symptoms associated with PMS like depression and irritability.[112]

Lastly, summon the girlfriends, ladies. We need each other. Battling through PMS is tough, but the compassionate ear of a good friend can do wonders. Do not underestimate the importance of talking it out. Your friends understand you. They're girls too!

Impede Insomnia

It is awful to want to fall asleep but you can't. It is even worse when the man next to you is snoozing soundly but you are still staring at the ceiling. Lucky us, women are more likely to have insomnia than men.[120] Many things can be the reason behind why you cannot sleep, including depression, illness, and stress. Lifestyle factors may also be to blame. So here's what you need to do. To help you get to sleep now, and every night from now on, read the section on insomnia in Chapter 5: Stress, Anxiety, and Depression, Oh My!

MIGHTY MAGNESIUM

This mineral is essential for managing PMS. You have probably noticed as you have read this chapter that it helps just about everything: bloating, cramps, menstrual migraine, weight gain, swelling of your hands and feet, fatigue, breast tenderness, insomnia, mood swings, anxiety, and irritability. It is pretty cool that one little mineral can do so much. But why is that? Magnesium is needed for more than 300 biochemical reactions in our bodies.[121] It is responsible for maintaining normal muscle and nerve function, keeping our heart rhythm steady, helping regulate blood sugar and promote normal blood pressure, helping us keep strong bones, and playing a role in turning fat, protein, and carbohydrates into energy, and helping support our immune system.[122] I guess if it can do so much, it is no wonder that it can help so much. If it is that time of the month and you are having trouble going to the bathroom (number two, that is) and/or you are cramping, these are tell-tale signs that you need more magnesium. Magnesium plays an important role in normal muscle contraction. It will help you treat the cramps you have, it will help you not get them next month, and it will help keep you regular too.

For those of us who need more magnesium to treat PMS, the RDA just isn't cutting it, and most of us are not even getting that much. Unless you are really paying attention and are regularly eating nuts, seeds, whole grains, and green vegetables, you won't ingest a sufficient amount of magnesium each day. Let's be honest. We really are not eating enough of these foods every single day, let alone the amount we would need to eat to obtain therapeutic levels of magnesium. The proof is in the pudding (which, if chocolate, contains some magnesium): large numbers (almost 70 percent)[123] of us are not even getting the recommended daily amounts of this mineral.[124]

Can you experience side effects from taking too much magnesium? Yes, but it is more likely you'll experience side effects from *not* getting enough. One side effect of taking too much magnesium is that you might have loose bowels.[125] (On the other hand, have you ever noticed that you are constipated around PMS week?) Magnesium citrate or magnesium glycinate cause less of a laxative effect.[126] They are very absorbable, as opposed to the not-so-absorbable magnesium oxide, a form more likely to get you running to the potty. The type of magnesium we choose is important for those of us aiming to take a bunch of it from now on.

Several factors affect decreased magnesium levels, including the intake of excess alcohol and salt, and the acidity of soda and coffee.[127] Did you notice that some of the items on that list are some of the very vices we use to cope with PMS? They also happen to be the very things we are asked to steer away from if we hope to treat our symptoms. Extreme stress, excessive menstruation, and diuretics can also drain your body of this much needed mineral.[128] This means that your magnesium approach should be twofold: reduce or avoid exposure to the magnesium suckers and take supplemental magnesium, along with calcium, because they work together.

Reduce the Red: Cutting Back Heavy Flow

It is no fun feeling like your insides are liquefying and gushing out between your legs. Besides cramps, having an overly heavy period is probably one of the most common menstrual complaints. Taking iron (about 15 mg per day) will help lessen your flow, as will taking extra vitamin C and bioflavonoids.[129] Women with heavy periods also have lower levels of vitamin A, and taking 25,000 IU of supplemental A has been shown to either restore bleeding back to normal or significantly reduce flow.[130] Vitamin E, in doses of 800–1,200 IU taken before and during your period also seems to relieve heavy bleeding.[131] As bleeding decreases during the cycle and in subsequent months, dosages of E are reduced, as are the number of tampons and pads you need.

IRREGULAR PERIODS

Is your menstrual cycle overly long, or way too short? Try adding 2–3 tablespoons of wheat germ to your daily diet. Mix it into yogurt, breakfast cereal, or use it as an ice cream topper. Wheat germ is a great source of magnesium and vitamin E, as well as protein and trace minerals. Many women report this simple remedy helps normalize their cycle and gets them right "on schedule."

IT'S TIME TO TAKE YOUR VITAMINS (AND MINERALS!)

You may think, "I don't know. Should I really be taking all of those supplements?" Do you feel better when you do? If so, then you have answered your own question.

There *is* evidence that vitamins can help alleviate the symptoms of PMS. Of course, there are sources out there that will be quick to disagree. You will be warned, cautioned, urged, and advised to really be very careful treating PMS or PMDD with vitamin therapy. If you want to fight this war against PMS without being just another hormonal casualty, know that vitamins work, and work well. They have a track record of safety that pharmaceuticals just cannot match. In fact, drugs do not even come *close*. According to the American Association of Poison Control Centers' report for 2009, there was not even one death

THE RIGHT PILLS FOR PMS

Let's be honest. If you are reading this chapter because you are "PMS-ing," then you are probably not in your most patient state of mind.

So if pills are what you want, pills are what you'll get. And these pills just happen to work well together because they are nutrients, not drugs. Here is a handy list to help get you started treating and preventing PMS with vitamins and minerals. Below are suggested amounts to take in addition to what you already may obtain through your food. Divide your doses and take with meals.

Vitamin A: 25,000 IU per day in the form of beta-carotene.

B-complex: Take one once or twice a day—look for a pill that contains 25–50 mg each of B_1, B_2, B_3, and B_6, and 400 mcg of folic acid (B_9); the amounts of B_{12}, biotin, and pantothenic acid can vary.

Vitamin B_3: When needed—take an additional 50–500 mg per day of nicotinic acid; or try "flush-free" niacin (inositol hexaniacinate), 500–1,000 mg per day; or take niacinamide, 100–500 mg per day.

Vitamin B_6: When needed—take an additional 50–200 mg per day.

Calcium: In the form of carbonate or citrate, take 1,000–1,500 mg per day; take separately from your iron supplement.

Chromium: In the form of chromium picolinate, take 200–400 mcg a day.

Vitamin C: 6,000–18,000 mg per day; take more or less as needed.

Vitamin E: 400–800 IU per day in the form of mixed tocopherols or d-alpha tocopherol; take separately from your iron supplement.

Vitamin D: 1,000–2,000 IU per day.

Iron: Take 18 mg per day in the form of ferrous fumarate, ferrous gluconate, or carbonyl iron; take separately from your vitamin E and calcium supplements. Too much iron can cause constipation, so if your supplement has more than 18 mg, just split the tablet in half, and save the rest for tomorrow or compensate for the extra iron by boosting your fiber intake.

Magnesium: In the form of citrate or gluconate, take 400–600 mg per day, or more as needed.

Omega-3 fatty acids: Look for a fish oil supplement that contains 900–1,000 mg total of eicosapentaenoic acid (EPA) and docosa-hexaenoic acid (DHA) omega-3 fatty acids. Read the label! A tablet that contains 1,000 mg of fish oil may only contain 300 mg of omega-3 fatty acids. You will want to take three of those a day to get the optimum dose.

Selenium: 55–200 mcg a day.

Multivitamin: Yes, you should also be taking a multivitamin. Yes, you should take it twice a day in addition to all the other vitamins and minerals you are now preparing to purchase. Look for one that also contains 15–30 mg of zinc.

from any vitamin or dietary mineral supplement.[132] And that's not just because 2009 was a good year. Over the last couple of decades, "poison control statistics confirm that more Americans die each year from eating soap than from taking vitamins . . . . Vitamins are extraordinarily safe."[133] How safe? Well, in the past twenty-seven years, there hasn't been one documented vitamin death.[134]

Some doctors push medication in the same breath that disparages vitamin therapy. When I was younger, this confused me a great deal. Why were doctors so very cautious if not downright discouraging about something as safe as vitamins, and so eager to tear a slip off their prescription pad with a potentially harmful drug scribbled on it? My father would reply, "Why would medical school doctors who study medicine and practice medicine and are heavily funded by pharmaceutical companies—why would they go look into vitamins?"[135] Medical doctors go to medical school to learn medicine and prescribe medication. The word "vitamin" just does not really fit in.

Though there is no cure for PMS,[137] if you fail to experience any

YOU AND YOUR AMAZING TECHNICOLOR URINE

You may notice when you start taking certain vitamins, or eating large quantities of vitamin-rich foods, your by-products start changing color. Even I was a bit shocked when I peed orange one morning. I did a frantic Internet search and then I took a deep breath. I realized my urine was orange because of all the beta-carotene I had ingested. (After all, I had drunk a quart of fresh carrot juice just hours before the potty "scare.") Though we have been taught, and rightly so, that the changing colors of excreted fluids is worthy of concern, don't worry yourself too much when it comes to supplements. Lots of folks comment that their urine will be electric yellow after taking B-vitamins, for instance. This is your body's way of dumping out the excess. This is normal.

"Wait, does this mean I'm just peeing out that pill I just paid for?" Some people think taking supplements merely manufactures "expensive urine." If a vitamin is excreted in urine, it means it has been through your kidneys. What has been through your kidneys has been in your blood. What has been in your blood has been absorbed by your body. Having an abundance of the essential vitamins and minerals your body needs, and getting rid of the excess, is good. It indicates that you have had enough.[136] It's deficiency that is a problem. Having a colorful bathroom experience isn't a bad thing when it comes to vitamins.

negative symptoms, then isn't that as good as cured? I know that what I have outlined here is not a one-pill solution. Combined with lifestyle and dietary changes, when you are taking your vitamins, PMS will have a very hard time holding you down. You have to learn about yourself and what you personally need. Take the time to find out what you have to do to be a better you, and do it. Then you may just forget that it is "that time of the month."

RECOMMENDED READING

Berkson, D. L. *Natural Answers for Women's Health Questions: A Comprehensive A-Z Guide to Drug-Free Mind-Body Remedies*. New York, NY: Simon & Schuster, 2002.

Hickey, S. *The Vitamin Cure for Migraines: How to Prevent and Treat Migraine Headaches Using Nutrition and Vitamin Supplementation*. Laguna Beach, CA: Basic Health Publications, 2010.

Hoffer, A., A. W. Saul. *Orthomolecular Medicine for Everyone: Megavitamin Therapeutics for Families and Physicians*. Laguna Beach, CA: Basic Health Publications, 2008.

Hoffer, A., J. Prousky. *Naturopathic Nutrition*. Toronto, ON: CCNM Press, 2006.

Prousky, J. *The Vitamin Cure for Chronic Fatigue Syndrome*. Laguna, Beach, CA: Basic Health Publications, 2010.

CHAPTER 3

YEAST INFECTIONS

*"There are a huge number of yeast infections
in this county. Probably because we live right
down the river from that old bread factory."*
—DWIGHT SCHRUTE FROM "THE OFFICE"

Let's face it, ladies: yeast infections *suck*!

We have enough going on within our bodies each month, thank
you very much. This just seems like a cruel, biological joke. We
should never have to deal with this. And it's not like after we have
one, we are immune from future intrusions; they can come back. For
some women, they do, and often. It's enough to make you want to
cut off your bottom half.

JUST WHAT ARE THEY?

Your vagina naturally has a balanced level of *Candida albicans (C.
albicans)*, the overgrowth of which causes icky yeast infections. Your
vagina can be a prime breeding ground for this fungus, especially if
things get out of whack: it's moist, warm, and dark. Bread rises better—and yeast is raised better—in just such a cozy environment.

Symptoms

What makes them so unpleasant? Well, if you have had the incredible good fortune of never having experienced a yeast infection (since three out of four women in the United States will, and half of these women will get recurrent infections),[1] here's the scoop: the intense itchiness, burning, irritation, redness, swelling, and copious amounts of icky cottage cheese-like discharge (eeww!) is enough to make anyone feel like they weren't so lucky to be born a woman. The discomfort and irritation alone can be so acute, it brings you to your knees and draws tears. Your doctor will know you have a yeast infection based on your symptom descriptions, and they may inspect your vagina and take a smear of the gunk to confirm the presence of *C. albicans*. You'll know beyond a shadow of a doubt that the next week of your life is ruined, and you will never eat anything that even looks like cottage cheese again.

It Gets Worse Before It Gets . . .

Wishing you could just have medicine beamed to your exact location, you stop fantasizing and go to the twenty-four-hour drugstore. Nonchalantly, you toss the yeast removal kit on the counter. As you try not to meet the inquisitive gaze of the adolescent chap at the register, you wonder briefly why you didn't just slip the darn thing into your purse and run for it.

Okay. Maybe your present embarrassment isn't worth the risk of being charged with petty larceny and landing in the police blotter headlining as the "Woman Accused of Stealing Vaginal Ointment." Instead, you focus on silently reciting the cost of the product, just in case he feels the need to call for a price check. You prepare to immediately and forcefully declare: "It's $17.49. If you touch that intercom I will kill you." Hurriedly, you hand him a coupon that saves you a couple bucks but doesn't save your dignity, and you wonder: shouldn't you have checked out with the kindly-looking lass three aisles down?

When the core of your womanhood is affected by illness, it is very hard to feel beautiful and sexy. You suffer in silence; the condition is downright embarrassing. You spend the next few days with gooey creams oozing out of you, making a point to avoid the "come hither" stares of your beau.

To make this whole process even more embarrassing and uncomfortable, television commercials boldly discuss feminine itching and infections. As you try to avert your gaze and hope your guy on the couch next to you doesn't start asking questions, perhaps you feel, as I do, an inner sense of equality when other commercials are broadcast about certain, personal, male conditions.

If you are lucky, the over-the-counter fix will be enough to cure you. Unfortunately, this is not the case for many women.

Now, before you go online and overnight a bulk shipment of yeast killer to your door (since you are certainly never going back to that drugstore ever again, even for toothpaste) do yourself a favor and keep reading.

Causes

Yeast infections are associated with a number of factors. You are more likely to get them if you have taken antibiotics, if you are going through hormonal changes such as menopause or hormone replacement therapy, if you are stressed, if you eat too much sugar and other simple carbohydrates, if you take an oral contraceptive, use steroids, if you are pregnant, or if you have diabetes. Monistat's own vaginal cream drug fact sheet indicates: "A yeast infection can occur at almost any time of life. It is most common during the childbearing years. The infection tends to develop most often in some women who are pregnant or diabetic, taking antibiotics, taking birth control pills, or have a damaged immune system."[2]

BIG BUSINESS

With an estimated 500 million cases of yeast vaginitis per year globally,[3] a whole bunch of us are going to experience a yeast infection at some time or another, and a whole bunch of us will turn to drugs to cure it. In the United States, it is estimated that over-the-counter antifungal therapies account for $250 million in annual sales.[4] In fact, antifungal drugs rank among the top ten best-selling over-the-counter products,[5] and that's just the stuff you don't need a prescription for.

Pfizer is the world's largest drug company. In 2002, sales of the Diflucan (also known as fluconazole, that one-dose prescription oral antifungal treatment) totaled approximately $1.1 billion worldwide.[6] In 2003, $1.2 billion.[7] Millions of people have turned to systemic antifungal treatments like Diflucan; I imagine numbers continue to rise.

Okay, I get it. Companies sell what is profitable. They're no fools. And hey, maybe it works. Maybe they make an effective product and that's why they are so successful. Yeast infections are *awful*. At least science is trying to help. Research attempts to show that medication works. The results, however, are far from encouraging.

The Bleak Outlook of Drug Treatment

There are numerous *candida*-killing azole-based medications such as itraconazole, terconazole, clotrimazole, fluconazole, ketoconazole, and miconazole. All of them are meant to target yeast overgrowth. For example, let's take over-the-counter miconazole nitrate (Monistat). If your immune system is strong, hopefully you can bounce right back to normal after this treatment. If you are fortunate, you'll also be spared any number of possible side effects, including abdominal cramping, headache, hives, rash, intense dizziness, itching, swelling, and trouble breathing, for goodness sake.[8] Yuck. (Antifungals can really make us anti-fun-gals!)

Even if you dodge the side effects, these drugs can create imbalances in their wake. *C. albicans* is suppressed (not eliminated) by such azole-based medications, and overgrowth of other non-*albicans* species can, and does, take hold for many women. Recurrent *C. albicans* vaginal infections are rarely due to resistance to azole-based medications.[9] In other words, if you have a yeast infection, it can be treated (at least temporarily) with an azole-based medication. However, the growing number of non-*C. albicans* species attributed to recurrent infections are intrinsically resistant to drugs.[10] Well, now what!? More drugs? One study suggested that a broad-spectrum antifungal is a possible solution to this problem.[11] In other words, let's kill all of the fungi. Even though this may seem to make initial sense, your vagina is about life and balance, not death. It would be great if you could just use one of these products and destroy only the bad stuff and keep only the good, but it just doesn't work that way.

One study[12] treated 387 women suffering from recurrent yeast infections with fluconazole, the active ingredient in the one-dose antifungal (Diflucan). They were given 150 milligrams (mg) every week for six months. After six months of treatment, about 90 percent of the women receiving the treatment were disease-free. Well, this sounds great, doesn't it? Only a sorry 35 percent of the placebo group had the same success. However, each group of women was monitored for the next six months without being given any additional fluconazole treatments. After twelve months, only 42 percent of women that had received the initial treatment remained disease-free. This means that *over half* of the women that used the drug just ended up getting another yeast infection within six months of stopping weekly treatment. The placebo group, admittedly, fared worse: only about 22 percent remained free from infection once the year was up. Two conclusions can be drawn here. One: doing nothing doesn't help. Two: taking the world's leading systemic antifungal doesn't help much either. Would we have to stay on the drug permanently in order to remain yeast-free? So much for the so-called "one-dose" treatment.

If you are suffering from recurrent yeast infections, I'm sure that you want a better than a one in two chance of getting another soon after six months of expensive, weekly, antifungal treatments. At best, azole-based treatments are suppressive, but they don't keep you from getting yet another infection. When you are on the drugs, you are not likely to get a yeast infection,[13] but "maintenance therapy" is not a cure for recurrent infections.[14] Fluconazole's side effects alone make you think twice before signing on to take this stuff for the rest of your life: nausea, vomiting, upset stomach, headache, hair loss, and allergic reactions such as swelling, rash, and severe dizziness.[15] Even fatal liver disease is among the culprits, not to mention lightened wallet syndrome.

Millions of women get recurrent yeast infections. Ladies, the question is: do you want to "manage" your yeast infections, or do you want to get rid of them?

That's a silly question, huh.

Conventional treatments for yeast infections can be messy, expensive, and ineffective, and I've found most to be all three. But here's the good news: each and every one of you suffering from yeast infections can treat yourself naturally and effectively without fear of drug-induced side effects.

Complications

Drug companies would have you believe that there is one pill, one treatment, one cream, one dose, one drug that can cure you. So you get a yeast infection. If you are willing to cough up the cash for treatment and deal with the potential side effects, you always have the option to go and face that fella at the twenty-four-hour drug store.

However, there is no guarantee that your symptoms won't come back unless you address what predisposing factors brought you this unpleasant yeast surprise in the first place. Have you recently taken antibiotics? Do you take the birth control pill? Is it the week before your period and are you pounding down sugar like it's going out of style? Pay attention to factors that may have set you up to get an infection, and be prepared to make lifestyle changes, especially if you start to experience recurrent infections.

Believe it or not, we aren't all that good at determining whether or not we even have a yeast infection.[16] Sometimes over-the-counter medicines are ineffective because the discomfort we are experiencing may or may not be caused by *C. albicans*. Abnormal discharge, if found to be caused by a pathogen, is more likely to be caused by bacterial vaginosis (BV).[17] BV occurs when the microflora, the healthy balance of good bacteria, is overwhelmed and outnumbered by the bad bacteria. This makes it all the more important to get a diagnosis first, especially if you intend to use drugs to treat your symptoms. Of course, I hope to convince you that drugs are not the answer. For example, let's take BV. The typical prescribed treatment for this condition is an antibiotic, a drug known to cause yeast infections. Hmm. Do you see a problem here? I imagine there are many women who suffer in this cycle of imbalance and consequential infections.

So, let's get this straight: even if you have an infection, there is no guarantee it is caused by yeast unless your doctor checks for it, so the medicine you buy for yeast might not work. If you know for a fact that you have a yeast infection, there are still potential side effects that can be experienced when using medication. If you know for sure you have a yeast infection and you successfully treat it with a drug, there are no guarantees that symptoms won't return, especially if there are predisposing factors that increase your chances of getting an infection. And if you do start getting recurrent infections, conventional treatment options are largely unsuccessful. As of yet, there are no real medical solutions for women who suffer from such recurrences.

Let's hear it again, ladies: yeast infections suck!

Well, I'm pretty sure you didn't pick up this book so I could tell you that medical options for treating yeast infections aren't particularly fabulous. You may already know that first hand. You probably were more interested in how vitamins and good health can cure your infection.

First, go to your doctor to get a diagnosis. Know what you are up against. Waiting to see a doctor is pretty awful when you are so uncomfortable you could scream, but as uncomfortable as you are, it is important that you know what you have. Knowing, for example, that you have a yeast infection rather than BV will help you take the necessary steps towards preventing a future infection.

The good news is, no matter what you are up against, better health will help you feel better.

IMPLICATION: IMMUNITY

Read this closely: research suggests that tolerance and immunity are the "only relevant defensive factors" against yeast infections.[18] In other words, if your immune system is strong, you aren't likely to get vaginal candidiasis. How do you create a more tolerant and immune vagina? You build a more tolerant and immune body. Build your immune system through good nutrition and vitamin supplements, and it will keep you free of illness.

Okay, sure. If I was healthier, you say, I wouldn't have a yeast infection.

Exactly. So let's get rid of the current infection, and then let's help prevent you from getting another.

WHAT TO STOP DOING

Many of us have probably heard of the basic no-no's: avoid wearing synthetic undergarments; wear cotton instead. Don't use scented or dyed toilet paper, or scented or deodorized tampons or pads. Keep the area clean and dry: for example, don't sit around in a wet bathing suit. Avoid powders. Avoid feminine deodorants. Avoid spermicide (nonoxynol-9) and lubricants. Avoid having sex until you are better. All of these are important, but there are some even bigger no-no's.

First of all, if you are on any hormonal birth control, stop taking it and seek out other alternatives. Women on the pill, patch, ring, or implant are significantly more likely to have yeast infections than women who are not taking hormonal birth control.[19] Yeast infections are more likely to set in just about a week before your period, and pregnant women are also more likely to get them. Why is that? For the same reason why hormonal birth control can influence recurrent yeast infections.[20] During certain parts of your menstrual cycle or pregnancy, estrogen hormone levels increase. Estrogen has been found to reduce the ability of your vagina to inhibit the growth of C. albicans.[21] It seems only logical then that women taking the birth control pill (containing estrogen) are more likely to experience a yeast infection. The birth control pill also weakens your immune system, the very thing you need to keep strong to fight off yeast. I have spoken with several women who, once they stopped using the birth control pill, stopped getting recurrent yeast infections. These same women experienced no difficulties with the pill for months after beginning use, but as months (and years) went by, the frequency and severity of their yeast infections increased until episodes were occurring every four to eight weeks. That, my friends, is no way to live. What is the point of being on a drug that prevents pregnancy when you don't have the chance to

So, I Can't Take the Pill Anymore. Darn It, to Say the Least!

I know what you may be thinking: "I do NOT want to get pregnant and...." I hear you: other contraceptive options aren't particularly simple or spontaneous. However, if you are one of the many women who are getting infection after infection, you are probably not having a whole lot of sex in the first place. So you have a choice: you can be on the pill, get more of those nasty yeast infections, and not have sex. Or, you can get off the pill, avoid infection, have sex, and find some other method of birth control you and your partner can agree on that doesn't cramp your style too dramatically.

have sex in the first place? Forgive me for being blunt, but it's hardly romantic to have a vagina that is itchy, red, painful, and oozing. If you are experiencing recurrent infections, I highly recommend that you take yourself off hormonal birth control.

If you take antibiotics, you are far more likely to get a yeast infection.[22] Antibiotics kill bacteria, but they are not selective. Both good and bad bacteria are targeted and eliminated. Opportunistic yeasts thrive in such an unbalanced environment.[23] Yeast infections stink, but antibiotics are necessary, right? Not always. In large doses, vitamin C acts as an antibiotic, but unlike an antibiotic, vitamin C will help your body target illness while allowing it to keep good, protective bacteria alive and well. Check out the next section for information about how to use vitamin C instead of traditionally prescribed antibiotics.

Sugar is not your friend. Alcohol is not your friend. Simple carbohydrates (like white bread) are not your friends. Artificial sweeteners are also not your friends. Sugars, alcohol, and simple carbs all cause a rapid rise in blood sugar and all feed yeast. You must *stop* consuming sugar. If you have a yeast infection, you may be particularly aware of your intense craving for sweets or alcohol. You crave it because *candida* craves it. Yeast rises best when it's fed, just like when you add sugar to bake that loaf of sourdough; the sugar you consume feeds yeast. If you deny the yeast sustenance, it will not survive. Reducing your sugar intake dramatically reduces both the incidence and severity of vaginal yeast infections.[24]

TO DOUCHE OR NOT TO DOUCHE

It *seems* like a good idea to "clean" our vagina, right? However, some studies show that douching increases your likelihood of getting a yeast infection.[25] The problem with douching is that you are messing with your delicate vaginal ecosystem. So, if all is well and good down there, it is best to leave it alone. However, if you already have a yeast infection, douching may help clear out some of the yeast you don't want. Vinegar and water or plain yogurt and water douches will increase the acidity of your vagina, and make it an unpleasant place for yeast to live.[26] Remember that your vagina is self-cleaning; washing it out, especially unnecessarily, may just make it harder to get back the balance you are working for.

Are you taking steroids, even short term, to treat arthritis, asthma, or allergies? Consider natural vitamin alternatives. Steroids are used to reduce inflammation and swelling, but a host of nasty side effects, like a compromised immune system and an increased risk for yeast infections,[27] comes with their use. Raw vegetable juicing and large doses of vitamin C can help. For more natural healing information about arthritis, asthma, and allergies, check out the books *The Vitamin Cure for Allergies* by Damien Downing, Ph.D., and *Doctor Yourself: Natural Healing That Works* by Andrew W. Saul, Ph.D., or go to www.DoctorYourself.com.

WHAT TO START DOING

It would be cool if our bodies were just like car engines. If something goes wrong, just go to that broken part and heal it independently from the rest. In many ways, this is what modern medicine attempts to do. It creates all sorts of specialized tools to fix specific parts, but often these processes have detrimental side effects, and the parts they attempt to fix do not always remain repaired. It is as if medicine puts black tape over the check engine light. That obnoxious light no longer glares at you, but the real reason behind why the indicator went on in the first place remains unchecked. In order to get rid of those dang yeast infections, you need to go to the source of the issue and not simply rely on a drug to suppress symptoms. It *is* possible to get rid of yeast without drugs.

Eat eight ounces of yogurt every single day, forever. The helpful bacteria you are ingesting in each bite not only help regulate your digestion, but they will also increase the presence of good microorganisms in your body, overwhelming the out-of-control bad bacteria. Daily ingestion of yogurt decreases your chances of getting a yeast infection and inhibits the colonization of *C. albicans*.[29] If you want to help prevent (and cure) yeast infections and you aren't putting down yogurt, it is recommended that probiotics be part of your daily regimen. Probiotic tablets, specifically ones containing *Lactobacillus acidophilus,* have been found to help build immunity against *C. albicans* overgrowth.[30] The good news is: it's hard to hurt yourself with a spoon of yogurt, even if you do drop it on your foot, and probiotics are just as safe.[31] Additionally, if you must take antibiotics, it is absolutely essential that you replensish good bacteria by contionuously reintroducing probiotics. It just makes sense.

Okay, now we are going to get personal. I have spoken with numerous women who don't just eat yogurt every day to overcome yeast; they also introduce it specifically into the infected area and have had positive results. Since I'm not one to be shy, here's what you do. Buy plain, unsweetened yogurt from the grocery store. Plain yogurt naturally contains some sugar, so don't be worried if you see some listed on the label. However, you'll want to avoid flavored yogurts because they have added sugar; avoid fruit and other additives, too. Dip in your index finger and scoop up a glob (a teaspoon or so) and put it right up inside your vagina. Do this at bedtime so the good bacteria have a chance to "settle in." Repeat this process for

WHEN YOUR WHOLE BODY GETS A YEAST INFECTION

Yeast doesn't just hang around in your vagina. It can show up in your mouth (also known as thrush) or on your skin in the form of a rash. Women who experience chronic infections may find that yeast has spread throughout their body; *it may or may not be visible.* William Crook, M.D., has written numerous books on the connection between *C. albicans* and numerous health problems, and Dr. Carolyn Dean, a naturopathic doctor and a medical doctor, has also spent years working with patients who have yeast-related disorders. Their checklist[28] for yeast-connected problems asks questions such as: Do you feel "sick all over"? Are you fatigued? Do you crave sugar? Do you sometimes feel "spaced out"? Do you experience depression or are you anxious or irritable? Are you bothered by headaches, food sensitivities, or digestive issues? Are you sensitive to tobacco, smoke, perfume, or other chemicals? Have you taken antibiotics or birth control pills? If you find yourself nodding along, you need to take a trip to the library and check out *The Yeast Connection and Women's Health.* To get started right now, you can go to www.yeastconnection.com for a chart to track your symptoms. Defeating a systemic yeast infection takes time and close monitoring of your diet and lifestyle. It is not easy to take control of your body once yeast has taken control of you, and it's hard not to feel discouraged and alone. You have to know that you can and will get better, just like so many other women have. For other helpful books, look for the "Recommended Reading" section at the end of this chapter.

a few days or until you see noticeable improvement in your yeast condition. Putting yogurt "down there" is enough to raise anyone's eyebrows, but many of the girls I know that tried it felt far more comfortable using a natural method to balance their vaginal chemistry than dealing with the drug-induced infection cycle they experienced with over-the-counter or prescription medications. Why does this work? *Lactobacillus acidophilus* (occurring naturally in your vagina and also contained in yogurt) creates an environment that is more acidic, a living condition that yeast doesn't like.[32] The best part is: inserting yogurt didn't cause any problems for the ladies that tried it. For some it stung a little, but it was not nearly as uncomfortable as a yeast infection. In fact, the only thing that really was harmed was their ego, as it was sometimes difficult to explain why they were heading to the bathroom with a dairy product.

Eat garlic and keep eating lots of it. If you happen to L-O-V-E garlic like I do, this is no trouble at all, except my husband would like to point out that the quality of my breath sometimes suffers a tad. An immune system strengthener, garlic's anticandidal properties[33] make it an easy to come by, inexpensive, and safe way to help treat yeast infections. Oh, and if you just can't bring yourself to eat it, try taking capsules instead: 400–600 mg twice a day.

Drink lots of water. Yes, that is still, and always will be, a good idea!

Try to de-stress. Uh-huh. That's the hardest thing to do on this list. Well, we still have to try. Stress decreases immunity; you may have noticed that you get sick more often when you are experiencing a great deal of anxiety or tension. If you need help de-stressing, try getting more exercise, try meditation, or some relaxation techniques, or all of them. If you are still feeling overwhelmed, check out the section on B vitamins. You'll be amazed at how well they work.

Keep an eye on your guy, too. For the most part, you aren't going to be having a whole lot of sex while you are treating an infection. It would hurt too much and it's kinda gross. If you find yourself getting better, and he has dry, cracked skin on his penis indicating a possible yeast infection (ouch!), don't jump back into bed just yet. There is little evidence to suggest that he's got anything to do with you getting an infection in the first place[34]—in fact it is more likely that he got it from you.[35] Treating him won't cure your infection or possible recurrences[36] but if he has one, it doesn't make a whole lot of sense to insert an infected organ back inside of you. Both of you need to get healthy before rekindling your physical love. Waiting isn't easy when you want to be close with one another, but hang in there. Do your best to get healthy, and know that your love life will be that much better when you don't have to worry about getting yeast infections!

A great way to build your immune system and provide your body with tons of nutrients is to start juicing raw vegetables. Don't knock it before you try it; juicing is one of the best ways to get yourself healthy and *feel* great. It is unlikely that you will down three pounds of carrots and a half a pound of beets (with a touch of cilantro for flavor) in one sitting. But that's exactly how much I fit into a pint glass that is adorned, albeit ironically, with a beer advertisement. I guzzle this down almost every morning—raw veggie juice that is, not beer. My mother lovingly named this beverage a "carrot milkshake" and though you may not fully believe her, I think you'd be surprised how good it actually is. I highly recommend buying a juicer (they cost anywhere from thirty bucks to several hundred) and some carrots for starters. Hint: take a bite of the raw carrot before you juice it; if it tastes good, your juice will too. Old bitter carrots make old bitter juice; sweet tasty carrots make sweet, tasty juice.

Drinking raw veggie juice has numerous health benefits. For example, beta-carotene, an antioxidant found in carrots, is a safe, non-toxic immune system builder even in high doses.[37] In your body, it converts into vitamin A, a vitamin known to help fight off infection. In women with vaginal candidiasis, beta-carotene levels are low.[38] Give your body what it needs by making a lifestyle change: start juicing regularly. Even though veggie juice made from carrots contains sugar, and some would argue that those with yeast infections should avoid such foods, remember that compared to processed, starchy, sweet foods, the sugar content of carrots is low. If you find yourself juicing a lot, consider mixing other items into your carrot base. Carrot-apple is pretty tasty, for example, and carrot-beet-cilantro-cabbage is my favorite. Be creative!

Some Other Natural Remedies

Here are a few other natural remedies for yeast infections. They are fairly easy to find. They can be located in your local (larger) grocery stores, especially retailers that have a natural foods section, or you can order them online.

Boric acid suppositories (600 mg; inserted at bedtime) are recommended for women who are resistant to traditional drug treatments.[39] This substance (as you can tell by its name alone) makes your vagina more acidic, and therefore less hospitable to yeast.

Other suggestions include taking the herb pau d'arco (and try 500 mg twice a day), oregano oil (50 mg four times a day), caprylic acid (1,000–2,000 mg three times a day) and echinacea, an immune system builder that may help make the body more resistant to C. *albicans*.[40]

PAINFUL SEX, AND RED, IRRITATED LABIA

Betsey's private parts were very irritated during intercourse. They were so red, sore, and swollen, and she didn't really want to continue having sex because it hurt too much. Sometimes, she would be red and irritated down there for no apparent reason. Other times, sex would cause the area to become inflamed when it seemed fine before. She didn't have a yeast infection as far as she could tell, but sometimes she noticed little white specks around her clitoris. She kept the area clean, so she knew it wasn't leftover lint or tissue. Thinking that her irritation might be related to yeast, she applied vitamin E mixed with one drop of pure tea tree oil to her inner labia, spread it all over the affected area, and went to sleep. The tea tree oil made the area tingle a little bit, but that was a far better sensation than the painful irritation she felt earlier. The next morning, her labia were back to their original fleshy color and she didn't much notice their existence. She decided that's the way it should be, unless they were otherwise summoned.

A large number of cases of vulvodynia may be due to yeast overgrowth.[42] Treating symptoms topically may help, but it is even more important that you build up your immune system so it can fight the root cause of your irritation. Healthy eating and taking vitamins can help you do just that.

Tea tree oil is another natural antifungal effective against *C. albicans*.[41] A drop or two diluted (to avoid irritation) with the contents of a vitamin E capsule or a small amount of olive oil and applied externally may give you some topical relief from your yeast infection. Tea tree oil is also available in suppository form if you want to place it right up in there.

Grapefruit seed extract is another recommended *candida*-killer,[43] also known as citrus seed extract. Once again, you'll want to dilute it before using it externally on your sensitive parts! Douching is not recommended if all is well and good downstairs, but if you are fighting yeast, douching with either a small amount of tea tree oil and water or grapefruit seed extract and water (1 teaspoon of either for every two cups of water) will help combat the yeasties. Taken orally, 500 mg of grapefruit seed extract three times daily is recommended.[44]

THE VITAMIN SOLUTION

There is no one thing you can do to cure any illness, just as there is no one thing you do to cure a yeast infection. Even remedies for the common cold suggest that you drink lots of water *and* get rest. It just makes sense to get healthy from the inside out and not simply rely on a medicine to work wonders.

Health is just not achieved by adding chemicals to your already over-taxed immune system. Health is achieved by providing your body with the vitamins and nutrients it needs.

Ideally, you would be able to eat enough of the nutrient-rich foods to obtain therapeutic levels of vitamins, but this is hard (if not downright impossible) for us to do. You should continue to eat raw fruits, raw vegetables, and whole grains in abundance. Do your best to avoid processed, refined, artificially colored, artificially flavored, chemically preserved, sugar-laden foods. If you don't know (and can't pronounce) the ingredients on the label, don't eat it. (I've often found if there is one bad-for-you ingredient, there are often several.) Vitamin supplements are safe, effective, and cheap, and they help provide in greater amounts the nutrients required by our bodies to cure illness, amounts that we may not otherwise be able to get from our food.

What Vitamins Do I Take, and How Much?

Start building your immune system with a good multivitamin. It is recommended that all adults take a multi to help prevent chronic disease.[45] Take two a day.

Take more C. Lots more. Vitamin C helps build your immune system so you can fight off infection, and it can take the place of antibiotics.[46] Antibiotics kill off bad bacteria, but they also attack the good stuff like *Lactobacillus acidophilus*. This is the very same bacteria present in your vagina that helps fend off yeast. So, the next time you get sick with a brutal cold and are on your way to fill a doctor's prescription for an antibiotic, try buying a huge bottle of C instead. Will it work? You betcha. I didn't take a single antibiotic until I went to college. It's not that I didn't get sick. I just had different tools to get well. Since we know antibiotics can lead to yeast infections, it just makes sense to try a safe and inexpensive alternative. You can always change your mind and go get drugs.

Vitamin C, also called ascorbic acid, is very safe. It is water soluble, so if you take more than your body needs, it is excreted in your urine. There is a huge amount of research out there that has shown for years how large quantities of C help fight and prevent infections and disease. How much C you need depends on one thing: *you*. The healthy intake for an adult can be anywhere from 500 mg to 20,000 mg a day or more.[47] You'll notice that when you start taking more C, you have more energy, your mood is elevated, you're less likely to get ill, and darn it, you just feel better. The best way to find out how much C you need is to get to bowel tolerance. In other words, if you take too much, you get diarrhea. This is not what we're going for, pun intended. The ideal amount of C to take is just under what it takes to put you on the toilet. So, to obtain a therapeutic dose, start with 2,000 mg three times a day. If you have a sensitive stomach, take it with food at breakfast, lunch, and dinner, or buffer your dose with a calcium-magnesium supplement. Gradually increase or decrease the amount of C you take until you reap all the benefits, but can avoid excess gas or loose bowels. You'll find when you are sick or stressed out you can take a lot of C without any side effects because your

---

WHAT BRAND OF VITAMINS DO I BUY?

It doesn't really matter what brand you buy. Cheap tablets can be just as effective as the expensive ones. It is a good idea to find tablets that are free of paint, other artificial additives, or fillers. Check the potency; sometimes it takes many tablets of one brand to equal the dosage in one tablet of another. Check the expiration date, too. Some vitamins, like C, also come in powdered form, which then can be mixed into your favorite fruit juice. This can be helpful (and less expensive), especially when taking larger quantities.

---

nutritional need for this vitamin is increased.[48] Help combat stress and keep your immune system strong by upping your dose when you feel overly anxious. Oh, and just in case you were wondering, I take 6,000–10,000 mg every day and far more (sometimes darn near 10,000 mg an hour) if I get sick.

Previously, I mentioned the importance of beta-carotene (vitamin A) and vegetable juicing. In addition to juicing, supplement your diet with vitamin A capsules, in the form of beta-carotene, especially on days when you don't juice. Vitamin A is an "immune enhancer,"[49] exactly the kind of thing needed to help strengthen your system. Getting your vitamins through juicing is ideal, but if you can't, taking a supplement works too.

If you are pregnant, the recommended dosages for vitamin A change, as large amounts of *fish oil* vitamin A can cause birth defects—but then again, so can vitamin A deficiency.[50] If you are pregnant, chat with your doctor before taking supplemental A, or just stick to carrot juicing. Beta-carotene (found in carrots, thus the similarity in name) is considered safe and nontoxic, even in large doses.[51] Beta-carotene converts into vitamin A in your body, and your body is smart enough to convert just the right amount it needs. The only weird thing that might happen if you drink a whole bunch of carrot juice is that you might turn orange. No, really! It's called hypercarotenosis, and it is completely harmless.[52] I drink a ton of carrot juice, and I have yet to look like a pumpkin. Even if you do manage to change color, it looks no worse than a fake tan. And just like those artificial self-tans, it goes away!

Vitamin E can be used topically to soothe irritated, sore, skin outside of your vagina. Taken internally, it is another immunity builder.[54] Suggested daily dosage: 400–800 IU. Look for natural E, d-alpha tocopherol, rather than dl-alpha tocopherol. That little "l" after the "d" means you are buying a synthetic form of E that is not as absorbable, although it is usually cheaper that natural E.

Let's hear it for B vitamins! For those of you who feel really stressed out, anxious, or irritable, get comfortable with the Bs. You may notice that when you have a yeast infection, you are overly touchy and tense. Little things can really make you mad, or really nervous and worried. Your mood swings may seem more intense than usual. Some symptoms of yeast overgrowth are anxiety, depression, and irritability, and conversely, stress can contribute to yeast overgrowth. If there are any vitamins you should start taking yesterday, besides vitamin C and a good multi, they're the B vitamins. For starters, grab a B-complex. Take it every day. B vitamins work best as a team, but when you are in the midst of an acute emotional episode, take additional B_3,[55] in the form of niacinamide. Suggested dosage: 500 to 1,000 mg. Or take extra B_6: suggested dosage is 50–200 mg. Start with the smaller dosage, see how you feel; then take more if needed. You'll be surprised at how quickly after taking B-

ZINC

This mineral stimulates the growth of T lymphocytes, cells that help clean up other infected cells in your body. If you are a huge fan of oysters, you are probably getting enough zinc. As for the rest of us, we need at least 15 mg of zinc each day,[53] the amount contained in a good multivitamin, but taking 20–30 mg is even better, and very safe. I like to take zinc with meals; otherwise, it can temporarily make me feel a little queasy.

complex and extra B_3 or B_6 your mood will even out. You feel like yourself again, ready and able to handle whatever was driving you so crazy before.

"Um, these amounts seem really high..." you say. Yes, but vitamins are really safe. And they are a whole lot safer than any drugs you are thinking about using to cure that yeast infection. If you want to really know how safe vitamins are, check out the article on vitamin toxicity entitled "Where Are the Bodies?" on www.doctor yourself.com or the numerous articles on the topic from the Orthomolecular Medicine News Service at http://www.orthomolecular.org/ resources/omns/index.shtml.

THE RIGHT PILLS TO TREAT YEAST INFECTIONS

Vitamins are an important part of a natural remedy for yeast infections. Remember to divide your doses and take them with food.

TO HELP TREAT YOUR YEAST INFECTION AND PREVENT ONE IN THE FUTURE:

Vitamin A: 25,000 IU per day in the form of beta-carotene, and drink fresh veggie juice, one to three pints per week.

Vitamin C: 6,000–18,000 mg per day; take more or less as needed.

Vitamin E: 400–800 IU per day in the form of mixed tocopherols d-alpha tocopherol.

B Vitamins: Take a B-complex twice a day that contains 25–50 mg of B_1, B_2, B_3, and B_6, 25–50 mcg of B_{12}, and 400 mcg of folic acid. Take extra B_3 (500–1,000 mg niacinamide) and B_6 (50–200 mg) as needed to help manage mood.

Multivitamin: Take twice a day in addition to your other vitamins and minerals; look for one that contains 15–30 mg of zinc.

HOW YOU FEEL AS YOU START TO GET BETTER

As yeast dies off (that's good!), it releases toxins into your body (that's bad!). These toxins will cause you to get headaches, feel joint pain, experience nausea, and feel tired and irritable.[56] As you treat yeast, especially if it has spread, you will feel worse before you feel better. This can be a bit disconcerting. You must tell yourself that you *can* get through this. You will get better. Do not give up. Drink lots of water and take vitamins C and E to help eliminate toxins. Take B vitamins to help elevate your mood.

BE YOUR OWN BEST DOCTOR

There is a whole lot of advice out there about how to cure yeast infections. Some is good; some is downright misleading. Be informed and be careful. Once you start looking, you'll also find plenty of folks ready and willing to sell you natural, specialized (and often expensive) yeast treatments and cures. Are they worth trying? You have to decide that. I'm fond of cures that are effective, easy to find, and inexpensive.

Don't take my word for it. There are all of those references to check out at the end of this book and some books that I recommend you read listed below. Don't forget to talk with your doctor, but don't be afraid to educate *them*. Only you know how you feel, and only you can take steps to get yourself better. What has been outlined for you in this chapter *works*. Stay strong, stay motivated, and go kick some yeast-butt.

RECOMMENDED READING

Chaitow, L. *Candida Albicans: Could Yeast Be Your Problem?* Rochester, VT: Healing Arts Press, 1998.

Connolly, P. *The Candida Albicans Yeast-Free Cookbook: How Good Nutrition Can Help Fight the Epidemic of Yeast-Related Diseases.* Los Angeles, CA : Keats Pub, 2000.

Crook, W.G., C. Dean, E. Crook. *The Yeast Connection and Women's Health*. Jackson, TN: Professional Books, 2005.

Gustafson, H., M. O'Shea. *The Candida Directory and Cookbook*. Berkley, CA: Celestial Arts Publishing, 1994.

Saul, A. W. *Doctor Yourself: Natural Healing That Works*. North Bergen, NJ: Basic Health Publications, 2003.

Saxion, V. *How to Stop Candida & Other Yeast Conditions in Their Tracks*. Minneapolis, MN: Bronze Bow Publishing, 2003.

CHAPTER 4

BACTERIAL VAGINOSIS

*"The worst thing about medicine is that
one kind makes another necessary."*
—ELBERT HUBBARD

A good friend and I once decided that when we girls have to go
through any vaginal disorder such as bacterial vaginosis (and we
still must be seen in public), we should wear t-shirts with the phrase
"out of order" in small, but noticeable, lowercase letters across our
chests. To no avail: even with clear labeling, we still must interact
with others. We are left to deal with our lives and be just as busy as
we were before, now with a lingering jealousy toward bathrooms, ele-
vators, and vending machines that are branded "out of order" and
are lucky enough to actually be left alone.

Vaginal issues are such a private matter too; we can be absolutely
miserable, but we can't appear that way to anyone. It would be easier to get the flu. We could just admit, "I feel terrible. I have the flu."
Nobody really wants to openly discuss infections *down there*. Just try
mentioning the words "vaginal discharge" at your next social event.
Faces will scrunch up, your audience will disperse claiming they have
to "go over there now," and your conversation-stopping vaginal
problem now might be good for something after all because you
finally get your wish and are left alone.

Well, I'm tired of *not* talking about this. Millions of women end
up with vaginal infections each year. It only seems right that we discuss it for at least a chapter.

67

JUST WHAT IS IT?

Basically, bacterial vaginosis (BV) is caused by a loss of our normal healthy population of bacteria (predominantly the *Lactobacillus* family of good microbes), which is replaced by other harmful, nasty kinds of bacteria: an overgrowth of *Gardnerella vaginalis* and other anaerobic species.[1] The root cause of this icky infection is still unclear, and symptoms may vary from woman to woman. Unfortunately, it can lead to other, more serious issues, like an increased risk of pelvic inflammatory disease (PID);[2] it's associated with an increased chance of getting human immunodeficiency virus (HIV) or other sexually transmitted diseases (STDs),[3] and it is a risk factor for preterm labor, preterm birth, and miscarriage.[4]

BV is no fun at all.

Symptoms

Let's discuss discharge, shall we? Women may report symptoms like abnormal vaginal excretions with an unpleasant odor; some report that this may have a fishy odor or be thin and grayish, or both;[5] some women may experience itchiness or burning during urination. But get this: *most* women will report *no* symptoms whatsoever.[6] You could have BV and not even realize it! This is why it is a good idea to get a diagnosis from your doctor if you are experiencing anything downstairs that is out of the ordinary. This is also a reason, among others, to get annual gynecological checkups to make sure you are A-OK. Don't be shy; get to the doctor and spread 'em. He or she will look at a smear of your vaginal discharge under a microscope, and confirm the presence of *Gardnerella vaginalis,* or better yet, tell you that everything is normal!

THE (DISAPPOINTING) DRUGS

Drug cures for BV have always taken precedence. (What did your doctor tell you to take?) The prescribed treatment for bacterial vaginosis is an antibiotic. If you choose to take one, you might get better, but you also might not. If you are hoping for a cure, you won't be impressed by the results drugs have to offer, so keep reading before you start popping those pills or using that cream your doctor prescribed.

You do have about a 60 percent chance of getting better with drugs.[7] Well, "D" may be for "drug," but that D-minus 60 percent is *not* good enough for me. If our kids consistently handed in papers that scored in the fifties and sixties, we'd probably be a tad concerned. Why do we accept these kinds of poor results with our health?

Even with therapy that is (somewhat) successful, women often get vaginal candidiasis, one of those wicked yeast infections, after treating themselves with medicine for BV.[8] Why is that? Current medical practice is to give an antibiotic such as metronidazole, also known as Flagyl, clindamycin (Cleocin), or tinidazole (Tindamax) to treat BV. Antibiotics are known to increase the likelihood that you'll end up with a yeast infection.[9] After taking the prescribed antibiotic, you may not have BV anymore, but you may have just exchanged one infection for another. Great.

Recurrent BV is a medical poser. Half of us who take medicine to cure BV will end up with another infection within the year.[10] Recurrences are due in part to the failure to re-establish normal vaginal flora after antibiotic treatment.[11] Current recommended drug treatments (more antibiotics) are ineffective at preventing recurrences, and even with maintenance therapy, relapses are common.[12]

If you are one of the many women who get recurrent BV, it is unlikely that drugs will cure you. Antibiotics kill off good bacteria too; the same *Lactobacillus* species that you need to flourish down there in order to restore healthy balance.

To make matters worse, the side effects of drug treatments for BV

ANTIBIOTIC ALTERNATIVE

Applied topically to vaginal walls, povidone-iodine has successfully treated patients with BV[13] and is regarded as a well-tolerated alternative to antibiotic treatment. Discuss this option with your doctor.

aren't pleasant either. Nausea, headaches, loss of appetite, a metallic taste, rash, stomach pain, dry mouth, diarrhea, and, as previously mentioned, yeast infections may occur with your use of antibiotic treatments.[14] In more serious cases, you could experience depression, cramps, itching, sore throat, fever, severe stomach pain, vomiting, vaginal irritation, pain when you urinate, lower back pain, menstrual problems, and abnormal vaginal bleeding. Allergic reactions can also occur, which may cause a rash, itching, swelling, dizziness, and trouble breathing.[15] These side effects have been described as "minor but unpleasant,"[16] but I would argue that if a side effect is unpleasant, it isn't exactly minor. The drug industry would have us remember: "Your doctor has prescribed this medication because the benefit to you is greater than the risk of side effects."[17] Okay, but wouldn't it be nice if we could treat BV naturally, without the risk of feeling even worse than we already do?

I'll bet that for many of us, taking a drug (especially one that is likely to be ineffective) isn't worth those "minor" adverse reactions, especially for those of us who must put up with them. Just ask the plethora of women who are venting their frustrations about antibiotic BV therapy in chat rooms, blogs, and discussion groups. Their testimonials are grim at best: few of these ladies are finding cures with modern medicine.

BV AND ANTIBIOTICS: THE NEED FOR PROBIOTICS

If you do decide to take an antibiotic to treat BV (or anything else for that matter), be sure to take a probiotic supplement, eat yogurt every day, or both, during and after the antibiotic treatment to introduce good bacteria back into your system. Antibiotics target all bacteria, good and bad. It is a good idea to continually introduce the good bacteria found in probiotics and yogurt back into your system to help reinstate your natural, normal balance of mighty microflora and help prevent opportunistic infections.

DOUCHING: DO OR DON'T?

Douching is associated with an increased risk for BV.[23] It messes with your normal concentrations of bacteria. Although it is nice to feel clean and fresh, that feeling can soon be replaced with the uncomfortable sensations that come along with unbalanced vaginal microflora. So, it is best to leave well enough alone. However, *when you have BV,* you may be itching to get all that glop out of there (pun intended). You may want to douche for several days with a mixture of yogurt and water and then following up with oral and vaginal probiotics.[24]

WHAT TO STOP DOING

Certain behaviors definitely increase your chances of getting BV. Anything that would upset the normal balance of bacteria can be cause for an infection, so douching is to be avoided.[18] Smokers are also more likely to get BV[19] as are intrauterine device (IUD) users or ladies who don't use condoms.[20] Having a new sex partner or multiple sex partners is also associated with BV. However, there are women who have never had sex who still get BV,[21] which highlights the unlikeliness of sexual transmission and explains why treating your male partner for BV does not increase your cure rate or reduce your chance of recurrence.[22] We just can't blame the boys for this one.

Keeping all of this in mind, the basic no-no's are as follows: Don't douche. Don't have unsafe sex. Don't sleep with a bunch of people; you are less likely to get BV if you are in a monogamous relationship. Don't smoke. Avoid IUD birth control. *Don't* avoid your doctor; if things seem off, get checked out. Sometimes you may experience symptoms that seem due to BV but could be signs of another infection instead. Don't be worried about getting BV from toilet seats, swimming pools, or from touching anything around you; you can't get it that way. Don't rule out the possibility that hormonal birth control or steroids, drugs known to weaken your immune system, are also contributing to your body's susceptibility to BV. Don't be in the dark. Know what your risk factors are and be prepared to make lifestyle changes if you want to stay free of BV.

WHAT TO START DOING

Doing your best to avoid behaviors that increase your chances of getting BV is a great start. You also need to build your immunity against infection. It is a two-step process: let's get good bacteria back into your system to fight the bad guys, and let's boost your immunity to help fight your current infection and to ensure the infection doesn't come back.

The Probiotic Plan

To get rid of BV, you need to restore bacterial balance. You do that by introducing good bacteria via probiotics, either by ingestion or by insertion into the affected area. The medical community has begun to change its perception of probiotics only recently, even though research has supported their successful use for over 100 years.[25] Species of *Lactobacillus,* those good bacteria, are starting to get a lot more attention as they show much promise in the fight against BV. Recolinization of the *Lactobacillus* species is being recognized for its capacity to cure vaginitis.[26]

In fact, *Lactobacilli* probiotics can be *twice as effective* as drug treatment.[27] Want to hear the best part? There are *no adverse effects* experienced by patients who have tried probiotics,[28] even those folks who have weakened immune systems.[29] Those results are far more encouraging than the results drugs have to offer, drugs that only work about half the time with the inherent risk of undesirable side effects. Additionally, probiotics do not increase your risk of getting an opportunistic infection, such as a yeast infection, like you can get after using antibiotics.[30] Inexpensive and natural, probiotics do no harm and are very likely to help. It's definitely worth giving them a try.

Some More Natural Remedies

Let's arm you with an arsenal of natural, proven alternatives.

HOW DO I BUY *LACTOBACILLI*?

You can find all sorts of probiotics on the market these days. Cost and potency is a factor, so it makes sense to read labels to see what you are getting. Though certain strains of *Lactobacilli* are indicated for certain health issues, most probiotic tablets are a combination of several. Basically, they are all good. However, oral *Lactobacillus rhamnosus GR-1* and *Lactobacillus reuteri RC-14* or intravaginal *Lactobacillus acidophilus* have specifically been shown to cure BV.[31] Many gals that know will tell you that introducing *Lactobacillus acidophilus* vaginally (via plain, unsweetened yogurt) gets the job done. Plain, unsweetened yogurt just happens to be about the cheapest and most effective way of getting *Lactobacillus acidophilus* into your system. You should be eating about half a cup of yogurt everyday; so if you aren't—start. If you want to spend the money on the fancy probiotic stuff advertised on TV, don't let me stop you. However, regular ol' yogurt is likely to give you the positive results you seek at a price you can handle. Read the label: only buy yogurt free of unnecessary fillers, colors, or other additives. If you intend to use yogurt intravaginally to help get a jump on curing BV, be *sure* to just use plain, unsweetened yogurt. There's really no need to put fruit up in there.

For folks resistant to antibiotic therapy, boric acid (600 milligrams (mg) a day for fourteen days, inserted vaginally) has also been found to be very effective against BV, even recurrent episodes.[32]

Garlic is great. Eat plenty of it. Fresh is best, but taken by tablet, garlic is still an immunity builder and a safe, effective, and inexpensive way to help treat vaginitis.[33] Well-known for its health benefits for thousands of years, its antimicrobial properties in particular make garlic a good BV butt-kicker.[34] Your breath may be a little stinky, but as side effects go, that's pretty tolerable. Use a little extra mouthwash and brush your teeth more frequently; your dentist will be all the happier for it.

BV AND PREGNANCY

We have enough to worry about when we're pregnant, but this is not to be ignored. Having BV when pregnant is associated with an increased risk for preterm labor, preterm birth, and miscarriage,[37] all pretty scary associations. Our pregnancy manuals inform us that our doctors will most likely prescribe an antibiotic for BV during pregnancy. It is unclear whether or not using antibiotics will reduce the incidence of preterm delivery in women who have BV. Some studies show that when women take antibiotics for BV, it helps prevent early delivery,[38] while other studies show just the opposite.[39] With the high failure rate of drugs, alternative therapies look all the more appealing. This is why some studies suggest that probiotic therapy is the way to go.[40] When inserted into the vagina, yogurt containing *Lactobacillus acidophilus* was shown to treat BV and prevent infection in pregnant women by increasing vaginal acidity and normal vaginal flora, creating an environment less inhabitable for bad bacteria like *Gardnerella*.[41] Eating yogurt and inserting yogurt vaginally is safe and easy and has no risk of side effects, and you and baby will be all the happier for it. Additionally, vitamin C (250 mg vaginally, once a day for six days) has also been shown to cure vaginitis in pregnant women and reduce their vaginal pH.[42] Vitamin D deficiency is linked to higher rates of BV during pregnancy,[43] as is iron deficiency.[44] Talk to your doctor about increasing your intake of D and iron. To maximize absorption of the iron you are already getting in your diet, take it with vitamin C, and take it at a different time of day than your calcium supplement. Calcium is extremely important during pregnancy, so don't skip it. Just change when you take it. Additionally, try to de-stress. Chronic stress is associated with BV during pregnancy.[45] Consider doing relaxation techniques and stress-reducing activities such as yoga, meditation, and exercise. Certainly, every woman is different, but my mother made relaxation part of her pregnancy to-do list. I was born after one hour and forty-five minutes of labor, and I weighed ten pounds two ounces. (Sheesh!) Stress reduction works, with side benefits, not side effects.

Tea tree oil has been used to treat BV[35] and some authors believe this works because the bad bacteria associated with BV are more susceptible to tea tree oil than the good lactobacilli.[36] Getting rid of the bad stuff while keeping the good stuff—sounds good to me! If this sounds like an option that could work for you, tea tree suppositories are available. You might also consider mixing one drop of pure tea tree oil with a 400 international unit (IU) capsule of natural vitamin E to use as a topical ointment to soothe red, irritated, swollen labia.

THE VITAMIN SOLUTION

Your body's immune system can demolish BV, but you need to take care of that system in order for it to do its job. Vitamins help you do just that. Spend some time in the vitamin aisle next time you go shopping. Read labels and learn: avoid additives and look to see how many tablets you must take to get the advertised amount of the nutrient. You'll see that inexpensive tablets often contain just as much of the active ingredient as more expensive brands.

Vitamins

For starters, you should be taking multivitamins every day.[46] It is an inexpensive and effective way to provide your body with a variety of essential nutrients.

Take vitamin A. Vitamin A gets an "A" for awesome. A powerful antioxidant and healer, vitamin A helps treat and prevent infection.[47] An increased intake of vitamin A may decrease your risk of severe BV.[48] You should be taking 5,000–10,000 IU daily, and more can be okay while you are treating your infection, but if you are pregnant or can become pregnant, you should discuss your intake of vitamin A supplements with your doctor first. The best way to get vitamin A in a natural, completely safe way, even when pregnant, is via beta-carotene.[49] Embrace bunny behavior, and down carrots like it's your job. Juice those carrots for easy delivery; drink a glassful every day or two. Eat plenty of green, leafy vegetables, and orange fruits and veggies like apricots, squash, and sweet potatoes. You can also get vitamin A as beta-carotene in capsule form, although it tends to be far more expensive than carrots.

Women with vaginitis are often deficient in B vitamins.[50] Vaginal issues can also make a girl quite irritated, and B vitamins help take you from feeling downright ticked to a calm, more subdued "I-think-I-can-handle-this" demeanor. Take a B-complex at least twice daily,[51] and more when you really need a chill pill. B_3 and B_6 also do wonders for those overwhelming moments. Take an additional 500 mg of niacinamide[52] or 50–200 mg of B_6,[53] and you may find yourself more capable of handling life in general!

Women need more folate. An increased intake of folate is also associated with a decreased risk for BV.[54] Folate is a water-soluble B vitamin that can be synthetically produced as folic acid, a chemical that has the same biological effect as folate. Foods that naturally contain folate include beans and other legumes, dark, leafy greens, enriched wheat flours, cereals, whole-grain breads, wheat germ, and colorful fruits and vegetables. However, heating, chilling, and storage of what we eat can reduce folate levels 10 to 30 percent.[55] Furthermore, even with the Food and Drug Administration's mandate that grains be fortified with folic acid, many of us will not consume the recommended 400 micrograms (mcg)—and more if pregnant—that we should each day.[56] Additionally, if you drink alcohol, it increases your need for folate.[57] Safe, effective, readily accessible, and inexpensive,[58] folic acid supplements are only a few bucks a bottle and can be located at almost any drugstore. If you are taking that daily multivitamin as you are supposed to, you'll be glad to know that most good multivitamins contain the recommended 400 mcg of folic acid.

Vitamin E is a powerful antioxidant, but it's especially hard to get disease-preventing amounts unless you eat enormous quantities of foods that contain it. Most of us do not get even get the government recommended amount of E,[59] just 22.4 IU for women over the age of fourteen.[60] In order to get 400 IU daily, the amount you should take to help treat and prevent BV,[61] you'd literally have to drink cups of oil. In the immortal words of an adolescent: eew! Go buy some E: natural d-alpha tocopherol is the best kind of E to buy as it better absorbed by our bodies. Applied topically, it can also be soothing to irritated labia.

Take vitamin C every day. Vitamin C helps heal tissue and boost your immune system. It also happens to be very safe. Start by taking 2,000–6,000 mg two or three times a day in divided doses with meals. While you are treating BV, you may find you are tolerant of even higher doses. Adjust your dose as necessary. Know that 20,000 mg a day (and more) is still safe for everyday consumption.[62] Pay attention to your bowel tolerance; the worst thing that happens when you take too much C is you get diarrhea, along with feeling generally bloated and gassy. (This is not always convenient, especially when at work.) If this happens, cut back the amount you are taking. When you are sick or stressed, your tolerance for C will go up. This is simply because your body *needs* more C when your immunity is compromised. Conversely, when you are well, you won't need to take as much.

Vitamin C used vaginally (250 mg for six days) cures vaginitis with nearly an 80 percent success rate while also reducing vaginal pH, making your vagina a place vaginitis doesn't like to take up residence.[63] Recently, another study was conducted that used 250 mg of vitamin C intravaginally for six days to cure bacterial vaginosis, and the authors concluded that vitamin C treatment is both effective and safe.[64] Some women may find that when the C leaks out, it can be irritating to the already sensitized skin of your labia. Topically apply vitamin E to create a buffer to avoid the sting you might experience while using C intravaginally.

Vitamin D deficiency has been linked to bacterial vaginosis,[65] so you need to make sure you are getting enough. Very few foods contain D naturally, but you'll notice that items like milk and orange juice are often fortified with it. Daily recommended amounts increase as you age, ranging from 600–800 IU a day.[66] It is safe for women, even those pregnant and nursing, to take 4,000 IU daily.[67]

Minerals

An increased intake of calcium is associated with a decreased risk for severe BV.[68] You should be taking 1,500 mg of calcium each day.[69]

Yogurt just happens to be a great way to get some of the calcium you need. This is just one more reason you should be eating it every day.

The United States Recommended Dietary Allowance (RDA) of magnesium is around 320–400 mg, an amount that is hard to acquire in your diet each day unless you are habitually eating foods that have relatively large amounts of this nutrient, such as spinach (several cups a day) or nuts (about five ounces a day), or at least ten ounces of halibut, for you fish lovers.[70] You'd have an interesting diet, to say the least, if you ate enough magnesium-containing foods to get the

THE RIGHT PILLS TO TREAT BV

Let's get rid of BV and keep it from coming back. Here's a list of the vitamins and minerals you'll need to help you do just that. Remember to divide your doses and take them with food.

TO HELP GET RID OF BV

Vitamin A: 10,000 IU per day in the form of beta-carotene, and drink fresh (mainly carrot) juice, a pint per day until symptoms are gone.

Vitamin C: 6,000–18,000 mg per day or more or less as needed.

Vitamin D: 1,000–2,000 IU per day.

Vitamin E: 400–800 IU per day in the form of d-alpha tocopherol.

B Vitamins: Take a B-complex that contains 25–50 mg twice a day of B_1, B_2, B_3, and B_6, 25–50 mcg of B_{12}, and 400 mcg of folic acid. Take extra B_3 (250–500 mg niacinamide) and B_6 (50–200 mg) as needed to help manage mood.

Calcium: In the form of carbonate or citrate, take 1,500 mg per day.

Magnesium: In the form of citrate or gluconate, take 1,000 mg per day.

Multivitamin: Take twice a day in addition to your other vitamins and minerals; look for one that contains 15–30 mg of zinc and 18–27 mg of iron.

TO HELP PREVENT BV

Vitamin A: 5,000–10,000 IU per day in the form of beta-carotene and continue to drink fresh veggie juice, one to three pints per week.

Vitamin C: 6,000–18,000 mg per day or more or less as needed.

Vitamin D: 1,000–2,000 IU per day.

Vitamin E: 400–800 IU per day in the form of mixed tocopherols or d-alpha tocopherol.

B Vitamins: Take a B-complex twice a day that contains 25–50 mg of B_1, B_2, B_3, and B_6, 25–50 mcg of B_{12}, and 400 mcg of folic acid. Take extra B_3 (250–500 mg niacinamide) and B_6 (50–200 mg) as needed.

Calcium: In the form of carbonate or citrate, take 1,000–1,500 mg per day.

Magnesium: In the form of citrate or gluconate, take 400–600 mg per day.

Multivitamin: Take twice a day in addition to your other vitamins and minerals.

amount suggested for BV sufferers (1,000 mg).[71] Supplements sure come in handy.

Important for immune function and healing, zinc is another mineral you should be incorporating into your diet.[72] If you like oysters, you are in luck. Just six oysters contain 76 mg of zinc.[73] The recommended daily amount of zinc is just 8–13 mg.[74] It is likely that your multivitamin has at least this amount. Adding a little more, for a total of 20–30 mg per day, would be even better and completely safe.

GETTING HEALTHY

Building immunity with vitamin supplements is great, and often necessary given our diet, but it is even better when you can get nutrients right from your food.

I am sure you have heard this before: eat more fruits and vegetables. Well, do it! The Standard American Diet (SAD) truly is sad: for the last twenty years, only about 30 percent of us have been ingesting the recommended servings of fruits or vegetables each day, and far fewer of us are managing to eat enough of both.[75] It's time to do your part; make these healthy foods a bigger portion of your diet.

Juicing is a great way to get those fruits and veggies you need in far greater quantities than you might if you were to put them all on your plate in solid form. Just a quick search on the Internet will put you in touch with numerous resources with tons of recipes. Recently I bought a juicer for only fifty bucks. It doesn't have to be expensive to get the job done, but it's no good unless you use it!

BV IS NOT FOR ME!

Having a dysfunctional vagina is uncomfortable, embarrassing, emotionally trying, and just plain inconvenient. It sure is hard to keep your spirits up when you have to deal with such a secretive, sensitive issue. It takes a whole lot of fun out of being a woman. But you can take control of vaginitis. You do not have to rely on drugs that don't work. You can try natural alternatives that are both safe and effective, and will also improve your health now and in the future. Take a deep breath and know that you *will* conquer this.

CHAPTER 5

STRESS, ANXIETY, AND DEPRESSION, OH MY!

"I try to take one day at a time,
but sometimes several days attack me at once."
—JENNIFER YANE

"Why can't you just relax?" "Lighten up!" "Chill out!" "Just be happy!" Yeah, right. It's just not that simple! Your feelings are authentic. There isn't a magic switch that just makes us "happy" any more than there is a switch to pump our bank accounts full of millions. If it were that easy, we'd flip the dang switch! Nobody really enjoys being stressed out, down, or overly anxious. Nobody wakes up in the morning hoping to have a *really bad day*. Life is tough enough on the good days! It's probably an unrealistic expectation to think that there is a quick fix for any of this. However, we can expect to make improvements, step by step, to get closer to our ideal, contented self. This is where lifestyle changes, diet, exercise, and vitamins can help.

STRESS, ANXIETY, AND DEPRESSION AND US

Anyone can be stressed out, anxious, or depressed. It just so happens that women are far more likely to be than men. It is also not uncommon for us to experience more than one condition simultaneously, for example, to be depressed *and* anxious. All those girl hormones coursing through our systems in tune with our monthly cycles affect us too.

Stress

Tired? Unfocused? Unmotivated? Irritable? Tense? Is your stomach upset? Have you been experiencing body aches and pains? Is your appetite decreasing, or are you eating everything in sight? Are you having trouble remembering things? How about headaches? Trouble sleeping? Digestive issues? Is your sex drive dwindling? Do you feel like you just have lost control? Are you presently reaching for a dry martini just so you can relax? If any of this sounds a little too familiar, it could be a sign that you are super stressed.[1]

Yes, we gals are stressed. Even though it's more likely that men may be assaulted, have dangerous jobs, or go to war, we still trump them when it comes to being diagnosed with oodles of stress. (Believe it or not, compared to the guys, we are actually about twice as likely to meet the criteria for post-traumatic stress disorder.)[2] If you are a gal with a full-time job and a couple of young kids to worry about, this probably doesn't surprise you much. You know full well just how stressful life can be!

Women are also more likely than men to experience physical symptoms due to stress.[3] That means we don't just have stress, we *feel* it. Over time, being stressed can lead to anxiety, depression, or both, as well as weight issues, heart disease, high blood pressure, abnormal heart beats, menstrual issues, and skin problems.[4] Stress is sneaky. It takes its time. It gets inside and starts gradually messing with our system. We may not even realize that stress is the reason behind our health issues. We may think our symptoms may be due to something else entirely. We may find ourselves trying to treat those symptoms when what we really need to address is stress itself.

Anxiety

We are also more likely than men to be anxious,[5] that feeling of being nervous, apprehensive, powerless, or fatigued. We may have a sense of impending doom, sweat, tremble, or feel weak. We may be having trouble sleeping at night.[6] Anxiety can also leave us suffering with headaches, irritability, tension, a lack of concentration, and tiredness.

We may turn to alcohol or drugs to try to settle down. If we have anx-iety we might also have other conditions like obsessive-compulsive disorder (how many times did you have to check to see if your car was locked?) or have phobias. Feeling anxious is uncomfortable and troubling to say the least. It's no fun to feel out of control.

Depression

Depression favors our gender, too. Compared to men, us gals are about twice as likely to get depressed,[7] and some one in five of us will at some point in our lives.[8] Depression can be caused by many things such as stress, tension, upset stomach, headaches, nutritional deficien-cies, poor diet, sugar, thyroid disorders, endometriosis, serious phys-ical disorders, even allergies,[9] as well as hormonal changes, major negative life events, and seasonal changes. (Ever hear of the winter blues?) Depression can also be a side effect of prescription drugs like hormonal birth control. Many symptoms of depression happen to be very similar to the symptoms of being really stressed out, including: insomnia, lack of sex drive, frustration and irritability, appetite changes and weight changes up or down, lack of concentration, fatigue, memory issues, mood swings, and aches and pains. Depres-sive symptoms can also include feeling a general sense of sadness and not being interested in anything that would normally make us happy. We might feel helpless, worthless, or overly guilty, or we may want to just give up on life.[10]

MANAGING AND MINIMIZING STRESS, ANXIETY AND DEPRESSION

Since both anxiety and depression can be side effects of being really stressed over time, we'll take a close look at what we can do to reduce stress, among other things, and subsequently help improve our moods.

Exercise

First on this to-do list is exercise. Don't sit there and tell yourself that there isn't time. It's so easy to find excuses to not exercise, even if you actually like doing it. Yes, no doubt our days are packed, but saving time for something as important as exercising is essential. You wouldn't question your need to eat food when you are hungry or drink water when you are thirsty. Why question your body's need to move? "I don't have the energy for exercise," you say. Even if you don't, *move anyway.* You will increase your energy, not deplete it. Exercise will help you improve your mood naturally by increasing the level of that feel-good neurotransmitter serotonin.[11] Doing nothing all day can feel more tiring than taking that walk or getting out in the garden. If it's winter for over half the year as it is where I live, a few ten-dollar exercise DVDs can really come in handy. Or, just put on boots and go outside anyway! Join a gym with a friend; or take your best friend, your hubby, to the bedroom to exercise your mattress. If your desire to have sex has suffered along with your increased stress level, check out the chapter on sex drive.

Relaxation

It is also important to take a break. (This does not mean you should avoid exercise. It means you should also find time to just breathe.) Mothers have told children for centuries to go outside and get some fresh air. It can be immensely therapeutic to just take in the outdoors. Practice some deep breathing while you do. Scheduling a massage or trying aromatherapy, acupuncture, or chiropractic may help you ease tension and body aches. A nice warm bath can do the same.

Laughter

Laughing is such good medicine. It's hard to see the bright side of life when you are so deeply entrenched in daily battles, but it does not take long to jump out of that trench, just temporarily, to relieve some tension. On a stressful drive to work, one of my favorite stress reducers is to think about the last time I heard or saw something really funny. I play it back in my mind and often end up with a smile on my face. Or, I literally force myself to smile. It feels a little awkward at first, but for whatever reason, it helps me feel less down. As silly as it sounds, pretend you are happy, and you just might start feeling that way! My husband loves to find funny videos on YouTube when he's had a rough day. In a few minutes, he'll be in hysterics and de-stressed. There is something about cats landing in awkward positions that just puts a smile on your face! Music, meditation, reading, and picking up the phone to talk to a good friend can all help bring stress levels down. "I don't have time for any of this," you say. If you don't have time for any of this, *it makes it all that much more important that you make the time.*

THE RIGHT DIET AND NUTRIENTS FOR STRESS, ANXIETY, AND DEPRESSION

If we are battling with stress, depression, or anxiety, we may find ourselves on a food or weight roller coaster. We might flock to buffets for comfort, or we might avoid meals altogether. When we do eat, we might be reaching for what tastes good to us, but might not be good for us. We may develop eating disorders or addictions. We may self-medicate with alcohol, caffeine, or sugar to try to boost our energy or just to try and relax. The food we choose to eat, or not eat, can have quite an impact on our bodies and our stress, anxiety, or depressive symptoms. If we are making poor choices, it's unlikely that we will feel any better. What happens then? We gravitate back to foods for a "quick fix," desiring to feel better right now, but we end up doing more damage than good in the long run.

Eliminating junk foods from your diet, like stuff high in sugar or refined carbohydrates, is a great start. The same goes for stimulants like caffeine and depressants like alcohol. These things may make you feel better in the moment, but can actually cause you to feel *more* anxious or depressed.[12]

Eating regular nourishing meals is also a must to keep your blood sugar from crashing (and to avoid the subsequent trip to the vending machine or that carton of doughnuts in the lounge).

The Need for Additional Vitamins and Minerals

Of course, proper nutrition helps ensure you are getting a wide variety of all the nutrients your body needs. However, even a well-managed diet can still be missing something. Recently, I read a weight-loss article in Reader's Digest that had me stifling guffaws when it suggested that folks *limit* their intake of broccoli and other cruciferous vegetables to two cups per day.[13] Yes, *limit*. Is *that* really the trouble with the American diet? Too much broccoli? Who is eating too much broccoli? Most of us can't remember the last time we ate broccoli. Well, what can we expect, really, since this article also highlights bacon as a healthy part of a low-fat diet[14] and is printed in a magazine loaded with thirty-one pages of drug ads (over-the-counter and pharmaceutical), including a four-page ad for the cholesterol drug Lipitor, immediately preceding the "better limit that broccoli and eat that good-for-you bacon!" ridiculousness.

Just for fun, do a quick mental review of what you ate today. Did half of each meal consist of fruits and vegetables like the government recommends?[15] (Any broccoli in there?) Getting our vitamins and minerals through our food is ideal, but let's face it, that's not really happening, is it? The United States Recommended Dietary Allowance (RDA) shouldn't be a daily goal to reach but rather a collection of intake suggestions attempting to limit deficiencies. Many would argue that these allowances are inadequate, and plenty of folks don't even manage to reach these very modest suggested levels.

"I Don't Need to Take All Those Extra Vitamins."

"I get the RDA of all my vitamins and minerals," you say. "I've checked!" Well, everybody is different. Just because one person requires one level of a certain vitamin to stay well and feel great does not mean that same amount will work for someone else. For example, if a gal works at a high-stress job, her need for vitamins rises because her lifestyle negatively impacts her body's capability to stay its healthiest. You need more water when you exercise; you need more sleep after an exhausting day. Doesn't it make sense that you may need more essential nutrients when you are stressed, anxious, or depressed?

Vitamins aren't going to remove stress from your life, but they are going to help you cope with the inevitable stress you'll experience. They can help build your immune system and keep it strong since stress can so significantly wear it down. The best all-around solution is to reduce stress *and* take your vitamins, and given that we can't always manage our stress to the extent we might like to, it becomes even more essential that we keep our body armed with nutrients to help prevent stress-induced health issues.

Stress and Nutrients

Stress really takes a toll on your body, and as it does so, your need for certain nutrients increases. Failing to address those needs means you'll be more likely to suffer the physical and emotional symptoms of stress. Adding vitamin supplements to your diet can help correct those deficiencies so your body can better support you through stressful times. For example, one study showed that a multivitamin-mineral supplement given to hundreds of people who were over-stressed significantly improved their stress symptoms after one month of use. The supplement consisted of a rather modest 15 milligrams (mg) B_1, 15 mg B_2, 10 mg B_6, 10 micrograms (mcg) B_{12}, 1,000 mg vitamin C, 150 mcg biotin, 50 mg niacinamide (B_3), 23 mg of pantothenic acid, 100 mg calcium, and 100 mg magnesium. Authors added that "the rationale for this combination is based on the functional interdependence of the various ingredients as well as on their metabolic and psychological functions."[16] This interdependence is why it is best to take a combination of vitamins rather than one in isolation.

When you are really stressed out, a daily multivitamin may not be enough. Extra B vitamins (you could double up on that B-complex), vitamin C (3,000–10,000 mg), calcium (2,000 mg), magnesium (1,000 mg), pantothenic acid (300 mg), zinc (50 mg), vitamin E (400 IU), and vitamin A (25,000 international units as beta-carotene) are recommended[17] each day. You may want to take even more pantothenic acid (B_5) for its calming effect on the adrenal glands: 1,000–2,000 mg per day.[18] Keep in mind that taking zinc on an empty stomach may make you feel a bit queasy, so it's best to have it along with food, or simply reduce the amount you are taking. Magnesium can have a laxative effect, so you should divide your dose (as you should when possible with all the vitamins and minerals you take) and adjust your intake of magnesium as necessary if you experience loose bowels.

Vitamin C

Vitamin C is especially important. When your body is under stress, your need for vitamin C increases.[19] Taking extra vitamin C can "reduce the deleterious effects of stress and help us withstand the inevitable stresses that we encounter each day."[20] Boost your mood and energy level by taking vitamin C several times a day in divided doses. Start with 2,000 mg or so at each meal. Of course, you can adjust your dosage up or down. Keep in mind: very large quantities of vitamin C (even 20,000 mg a day or more) are not dangerous.[21] Did you know that in nature practically every animal can manufacture more vitamin C in their bodies when they are under stress?[22] We, however, cannot. That makes it all the more important to bolster our diets with extra C. Some would argue that when it comes to vitamin C, the quantity recommended by the RDA is wholly inadequate. Adjusted for body weight, the RDA would have us believe that we need 10 to 100 times *less* vitamin C than almost any other animal on earth.[23] This just doesn't seem to make much sense. Maybe they experience more stress that we do. I guess if I was lower in the food chain I might feel a little under pressure too.

I take what some would consider quite a lot of vitamin C. Normally, I take about 6,000–10,000 mg of vitamin C each day to maintain optimal health. But, when my body is fighting off illness, fatigue, coping with stress, or anything that takes a toll on my immune system, I might load up on vitamin C at a rate of about 5,000–10,000 mg an hour (yes, hour) in divided doses. Once I get to saturation of C (loose bowels), or preferably just before that point, I throttle and eventually I work back to my maintenance dose of about 6,000–10,000 mg total a day. How do I know how much to take? I listen to my body. If I am symptom-free and I feel good, I know I'm getting enough.

Depression and Nutrients

For some folks, depression may be linked to their need for certain nutrients. Low levels of certain B vitamins have been linked to mood disorders. For starters, low levels of folate (B_9) may be associated with symptoms of depression.[24] Low levels of this nutrient alone, or in combination with B_6, B_{12}, and vitamin C deficiency, may also be associated with feeling down.[25] For women with depressive symptoms associated with premenstrual syndrome (PMS), doses of B_6 up to 100 mg per day showed a significant benefit.[26] B_1 is another goodie. Two months of supplementation with 50 mg per day of B_1 helped women in one study feel "more composed, clearheaded, and energetic."[27] If you have depressive tendencies, you'll want to add a B-complex vitamin to your diet. The Bs need each other to do their best, so a B-complex (with additional amounts of specific B vitamins for your unique needs) is a great place to start.

Ah, sunshine. It just has a happy feel to it, does it not? It's kind of neat that our association between sun and happiness has a scientific connection, too. Vitamin D, the same vitamin your body manufactures when you are in the sun's rays, can help you be less depressed.[28] If you can't locate the sun in your area (perhaps do you live in cloudy Western New York?) supplements may be necessary to keep the blues away.

If you head to the fridge for mood-enhancing, quick-to-get-your-blood-sugar-up substances, you may want to take chromium picolinate to help level out blood sugar highs and lows. You may find that 400–1,000 mcg per day helps reduce overeating and reverse feelings of depression.[29]

The omega-3 fatty acids,[30] zinc, magnesium,[31] and selenium[32] are depression fighters.[33] Calcium may also be significantly beneficial for our moods. For example, 1,200 mg per day of calcium has been shown to help alleviate depression, mood swings, and irritability in women who suffer with PMS.[34]

Don't forget multivitamins! One study demonstrated that after a year of taking a high-potency multivitamin supplement, women reported significantly improved moods.[35] Since multivitamins contain all sorts of good-for-you ingredients conveniently condensed into one little tablet, those of you new to the vitamin cure world may want to begin by taking these. You'll "cover your bases," so to speak, by giving your body a wide range of essential nutrients—nutrients that are often interdependent and, therefore, increasingly beneficial when taken together. Then, if you find you would benefit from taking more of a particular vitamin or mineral, you add that on to the foundation of nutrients already present in your multi. Taking a multivitamin is kind of like putting on your undies every day. It's a great way to cover *your* base with an essential garment. The additional clothes that make up the rest of the outfit, just like the extra amounts of vitamins you take in addition to your multi, may change just as the weather does. Sometimes, you may need to really "bundle up" and take a whole bunch of extra vitamins to deal with a stress storm; other days, you'll just "wear something light" finding that smaller maintenance doses of vitamins do just fine. Be as confident taking your vitamins as you are when you put a winter coat on if it's snowing out: it makes sense, so you wear it! If you need additional vitamins to feel better, take them!

Foods rich in omega-3s, magnesium, and B vitamins should be on the menu. How much of your diet contains foods like beans, nuts (like cashews and almonds), flax seed, fish, and spinach?

Does all this mean you should toss out your antidepressants and jump cold turkey into a vitamin regimen? Not necessarily. Nutrition may indeed be the key to help ease depressive symptoms, but medication may still be required for some. No matter what, eating a good diet and supplementing with vitamins and minerals is worth doing. For instance, if you already take medication for depression, folic acid and other B vitamins may be a beneficial adjunct therapy to help the antidepressants work better.[36] Conversely, not enough of a nutrient, folic acid for example, could reduce your antidepressant's effectiveness.[37]

Anxiety and Nutrients

Do you ever feel anxious only to find yourself feeling *more* anxious because you're feeling anxious? You get that rush of adrenaline in your chest, you know you are feeling panicked, but it just makes it worse to know you should be calm but you're not. I've just described my typical drive to work. For example, one idiot pulls a crazy move on the highway, resulting in an adrenaline rush for yours truly. Now my panic response is disproportionally touchy, so every subsequent event on the road (deserving of panic or not) causes the adrenaline response once more. This feeling isn't necessarily reserved for some erratic driver either. Thinking about a stressful meeting, a confrontational situation, or just the incredible list of to-do's that I repeat over and over in my head until I get a chance to write them down; all can send that rush of adrenaline surging through at an increasing intense pace. I know I'm anxious, and then I feel even more anxious because I know that feeling isn't good for me and will wear me out. Sometimes deep breathing can help; sometimes thinking of something other than that anxious feeling can distract from the present. Sometimes, nothing seems to work. That when vitamins become really helpful.

If you are feeling apprehensive and panicked, you may want to consider looking into the benefits of B_3. Niacinamide is the form of B_3 "most effective for the treatment of anxiety disorders."[38] It has "therapeutic effects similar to benzodiazepines," the drugs most often prescribed to reduce anxiety (which they do), but niacinamide does not have all of the negative side effects.[39] However, all forms of niacin will be helpful for managing your anxiety.[40] If you are interested in learning more about niacin therapy for anxiety, depression, and other mood disorders, I would highly suggest that you look into the work of Abram Hoffer, M.D., who pioneered the use of high-dose niacin therapy. Several of his books are mentioned in the recommended reading section of this chapter. As for other helpful B vitamins like B_1, B_6, and B_{12}, they are easily obtained in a B-complex supplement. They are also going to be useful for decreasing anxiety.[41]

Minerals can minimize anxiety, too. Carolyn Dean, M.D., N.D., describes magnesium as her favorite mineral, and it probably should be your favorite too if you are trying to manage your anxiety. She explains, "Prolonged psychological stress raises adrenaline, the stress hormone, and results in a myriad of metabolic activities, all of which require and therefore deplete magnesium. Magnesium depletion itself stresses the body, which can result in panic attacks, which results in more bursts of adrenaline and creates irritability and nervousness. Not only do our overworked adrenals cause magnesium depletion, but even more adrenaline is released under stress when magnesium levels are low in the body. It's the proverbial catch-22."[42] Dosage-wise, start supplementing with at least 400 mg of magnesium daily in divided doses.[43] Dean points out that the RDA is around 350 mg a day, an amount that magnesium researchers find is not nearly enough. She recommends doubling or even tripling that dose of magnesium.[44]

Inositol, included in the B vitamin family, is another antianxiety nutrient. It has been shown to be effective for treatment of obsessive-compulsive disorder, depression, and panic.[45] One study that compared this natural alternative to the antianxiety medicine fluvoxamine, found that supplementation with 18 grams per day of inositol was significantly more effective than the drug at reducing the number of panic attacks paitents experienced.[46] Hmm. A natural option that is

KNOW ABOUT NIACIN (B$_3$)

There are basically three kinds of niacin: niacin (which is nicotinic acid), niacinamide (uncommonly known as nicotinamide), and inositol hexaniacinate (also called inositol hexanicotinate). Okay, that's fine; there are three forms of B$_3$. Got it. But . . . then you'll see niacin labeled "no-flush" and "flush-free" and "sustained-release" or "timed-release." More importantly, you'll read that one type of niacin is better for this or that over another type of niacin. How do you know which one is what? How do you know which one to take? Which one is best for what you want it for? It can be very confusing.

In *Niacin: The Real Story*, you can read about niacin in all of its glory. You'll read about how incredibly effective niacin is, backed up by lots of research. Hoffer, Saul, and Foster do a nice job explaining the types of niacin and their benefits in the first chapter. I'll briefly outline their description of the different varieties and what they are good for to clear up any confusion you may have.

potentially more effective than a drug, and it comes without the long list of side effects? Sounds like something worth trying! Inositol is available in powder or tablet form. B-complex vitamins usually contain a small amount, about 50 mg or so. To achieve very high doses, inositol powder is the better way to go. You'd have to take a handful of inositol tablets (at 500 mg each) to get the amount they are talking about in that study, whereas in powder form, you can get approximately 2 grams per teaspoon. If your symptoms aren't obsessive-compulsive disorder severe, you could opt to take far less and see how you feel.

Improve your mood and decrease anxiety? Selenium may be what you need. Folks with lower levels of selenium in their diet report more anxiety, depression, and tiredness, symptoms that decreased after taking 100 mcg per day of selenium for five weeks.[47] Selenium works well with vitamin E, so it's a good idea to take those two together.

Nicotinic Acid

Plain ol' niacin is also known as nicotinic acid. It isn't generally referred to as such because the name sounds confusingly similar to the word nicotine. Niacin has nothing physiologically in common with nicotine, but it can be helpful to know this "official" name when you are reading labels so you can distinguish between different forms of niacin. Nicotinic acid lowers bad, low-density lipoprotein (LDL) cholesterol, and is very effective at increasing good, high-density lipoprotein (HDL) cholesterol. It also "lowers triglycerides, lowers Lipo A [lipoprotein(a)], lowers the anti-inflammatory factor C-reactive protein and therefore is the best substance known for these important therapeutic effects."[48] It has psychiatric benefits, like improving mood or reducing anxiety. It generally does not cause nausea, even in doses of several thousand milligrams a day. However, niacin can cause you to experience a flush, a feeling of being warm, tingly, and even itchy, which some folks don't like. Taking less can sidestep the problem, and so can taking your niacin with vitamin C, but there are other forms of niacin to try for those who want to avoid a flush altogether.

Niacinamide

Niacinamide will not help reduce cholesterol. However, this form of niacin can reduce anxiety and can also alleviate arthritis. At high doses, niacinamide can cause nausea, but in *Niacin: The Real Story* Hoffer, Saul, and Foster point out that William Kaufman, M.D., used high doses of niacinamide to treat patients with arthritis and reported virtually no side effects.

Inositol Hexaniacinate

This form of niacin is very unlikely to cause flushing, nausea, or any other side effects. It is effective for mood disorders and it does have blood lipid benefits, but it is not as effective as nicotinic acid. Inositol hexaniacinate is sometimes referred to as "flush-free," "no-flush," "sustained-release," or "timed-release" niacin. Be sure to read the label. These various titles could also refer to a timed-release form of nicotinic acid. If you are looking specifically for inositol hexaniacinate, flip that bottle over and make sure that is the active ingredient. Why? If you take a sustained-release or timed-release form of nicotinic acid instead, you may find it distressing because these tablets can be "felt it in the stomach."[49] Additionally, it also may fail to break down in the digestive tract, reducing the dose of niacin you actually get. Hoffer, Saul, and Foster say sustained-release or timed-release niacin "is a perfectly good idea: If a vitamin tablet dissolves slowly, there is a sustained-release effect. This means a reduced niacin 'flush'. . . . But the biggest reason to avoid sustained-release niacin is that relatively more reports of side effects stem from use of that form. . . . We therefore prefer and recommend manual, regular doses, not sustained release."[50]

MANAGING SYMPTOMS OF STRESS, ANXIETY, AND DEPRESSION

Can't sleep? Got a headache? Are you fatigued? Achy? Let's get into what you can do to manage some common symptoms of stress, anxiety, and depression.

Headaches

Guess what? Women are more likely to get headaches than men.[51] (You're telling me, right?) Since we are more likely to be stressed out, anxious, or depressed, I guess it makes sense that we would be the ones getting the migraines. And there's more bad news. If stress is causing your headaches (or making them worse) there's really only one way to get better: get rid of excess stress. If you are suffering through a migraine or two every month, this is no way to live. You have a choice: you can reduce stress and actually enjoy more of your days, or you can keep pushing ahead at the same reckless pace and accept that migraines are going to be a regular part of your life. It's likely that once the headaches get bad enough, you'll find yourself willing to do anything to make them better. Admittedly, it would be better not to get to that point.

While you are working on reducing stress with such things like exercise, relaxation techniques, and schedule modification, there are other simple things you can do to help your headaches. For one, make sure you are drinking enough water. If you feel the start of a headache coming on, try immediately drinking at least a glass or two. It certainly won't hurt you. Then, make a point to increase your daily intake of water. Frequent-headache sufferers who increased their intake of water by about two and a half pints a day reduced the number of hours spent with a headache and headache intensity.[52] More water may be just what your body needed.

Are you one of those people who enjoys a daily cup of coffee or two when you're at work only to wake up on Saturday morning with a headache? Caffeine-withdrawal headaches are real.[53] For that reason, you may want to adjust your caffeine intake. You might have noticed that when you have more caffeine, your headache actually goes away. (Caffeine happens to be an ingredient in the popular over-the-counter headache medication Excedrin.) If so, I guess you have to ask yourself this question: if caffeine is the reason you get headaches in the first place, do you want to keep relying on it to fix the problem it's causing? Does it get to decide when you can and cannot feel good? Break the caffeine-headache-caffeine go-around by weaning yourself off that need for your daily cups of Joe.

A series of visits to the chiropractor may help. Some folks will find relief from their tension headaches with a chiropractic adjustment, avoiding the need to take medication. A hot or cold compress is another med-free tactic to try. Massages can work wonders, too.

Your severe headache could be linked to your body's need for more vitamins or minerals. For example, magnesium deficiency may be linked to migraines.[54] Other nutrients like vitamin D, calcium, omega-3 fatty acids, vitamin C, chromium, and the B vitamins (such as riboflavin, B_2[55] and niacin, B_3[56]) may also help you fend off that headache.[57]

Fatigue

Zero energy and zero motivation? Chalk it up to fatigue. Stress can really wear you down, and feeling completely drained is a common result. We're not talking about the normal tiredness you might experience after a physically strenuous activity; this is an exhaustion that lingers and weighs you down, making you feel like you have no get-up-and-go. Yes, it's possible that you need more time for rest and relaxation, but it's also likely that nutrient imbalances are to blame.

Here's a list of some things to investigate as you work on conquering fatigue:

1. Are you getting enough iron? The most common symptom of iron deficiency is fatigue,[58] and since you are a lady, it's likely you aren't getting the amount you need.[59] Take an iron supplement each day (18–27 mg) that contains ferrous fumarate, ferrous gluconate, or carbonyl iron.

2. Vitamin C helps your body absorb iron, so that's one good reason to take it. It also can fend off fatigue.[60]

3. B-complex vitamins help fight fatigue.[61]

4. Extra magnesium may improve your energy level.[62]

5. Zinc, selenium, and omega fatty acids may also be helpful.[63]

6. Make sure you are drinking enough water.

7. Evaluate if caffeine withdrawal is causing your energy level to crash. I know, if you are tired, caffeine is a solution, not a problem, right? Well, not really. It may be temporarily hiding your symptoms, but it's not helping the cause.

Memory Problems

My husband and I find lecithin to be especially helpful for getting rid of that fuzzy brain feeling. He will blend lecithin granules into a tasty fruit and yogurt smoothie in the morning. If there are other plans for breakfast, a dry tablespoon full followed by a gulp of water to swallow it down works nicely too—don't chew unless you want to tongue it off your teeth all day. I don't mind the flavor, usually described as "nutty," but if you do, there are plenty of ways to hide it in your food or you can just cave and take the tablets instead. You may just find that lecithin helps your memory. Of course, if you forget to take the lecithin . . . .

Insomnia: I Need to Sleep But I Can't Sleep!

It is an awful feeling to be lying in bed at night with our thoughts racing, knowing that we need to sleep, and we can't. Each minute, each hour that passes, we glance at the clock, aware that now we'll only get six hours of sleep . . . then five . . . then four. . . . This just increases our anxiety and we continue to lie there, awake. The next day we are exhausted. We just want to sleep. We need to sleep. But we can't.

It seems so strange that the very thing our body needs to relieve stress is the very thing we can't do when we are overstressed. We want to sleep so we can relax, but we have to be relaxed in order to sleep. Yes, we know full well that we need to find ways to lessen the stress we are feeling each day, but that knowledge isn't going to help us at 3:00 A.M. when we can't get the rest we need *now*. Here's what can be done now (and tomorrow) to help get a better night's sleep:

1. If you are a caffeine drinker, start to eliminate it from your diet.[64] Even that afternoon coffee you had hours ago could be impacting the sleep you aren't getting tonight.

2. Alcohol may help you pass out, but you are more likely to sleep lightly and wake up when you don't want to. Skip the drink before bed.

3. Start exercising. I know, if it is the middle of the night and your mind just won't quit, it is a bit late to be thinking about the exercise you should have done earlier. However, folks who work out regularly (and do so well before bedtime) will tell you that they sleep better when they are all tuckered out. Instead of drugging yourself to sleep, set a goal to get up and move more during the day. You just may find that exercise will help improve your sleep habits.[65]

4. Consider meditation to calm and relax your body and mind.

5. Make your bedroom a place for sleep. Block out as much light as possible, take out the TV or computer, and put your pet in another room. There's no need for any distraction when what you really need is some shut-eye.

6. Do leg cramps or muscle spasms bother you at night? You may need more magnesium. There may be a connection between low levels of magnesium and shallower sleep and waking up more at night.[66]

7. Not getting enough iron may be related to sleep and sleep disturbances.[67] Oddly enough, not enough iron can cause fatigue, but not enough iron can also make it difficult to sleep.

8. Some folks find it is easier to go to sleep if they take 3–6 mg of melatonin an hour before bed.[68]

9. Eating foods high in L-tryptophan may help you get to sleep at night and feel more rested in the morning. L-tryptophan is an essential amino acid that converts into serotonin. Milk, cheese, yogurt (along with carbohydrates like crackers or bread) chicken, seafood, beans, and cashews are all foods high in L-tryptophan.[69]

10. Niacin (B_3) in the form of nicotinic acid can also quiet your mind
    and help you go to sleep.[70] Take 50–100 mg or even a little less.
    (You can just slice a tablet into sections to get a small but approx-
    imate dose.) Keep in mind that how much you will need may
    change. When I am super stressed and my thoughts just won't
    quiet down, I can take up to about 500 mg before I get that
    sleepy feeling. Other nights, 50–100 mg will do. My husband
    takes anywhere from 100–500 mg. We take the smaller amount
    right before bed, and then take a little more if we do not get that
    calming feeling within thirty minutes or so. You may find you are
    sleeping before you get a chance to figure out if it is working.
    Nicotinic acid may cause you to look flushed and feel itchy or
    even nauseous. This may not sound very pleasant, but a small
    amount of flushing may feel warm and calming to you. The expe-
    rience is more intense if you have taken a larger amount, espe-
    cially on an empty stomach, and that's why it is best to start small
    to avoid a really strong reaction. Over time, you will find that
    you can take a little more niacin and not experience the same ini-
    tial flushing intensity you felt when you first started taking the
    vitamin. Flushing is a histamine reaction and is harmless,[71]
    although some folks find it unnerving. You may prefer to take the
    flush-free variety of niacin, inositol hexaniacinate, to avoid the
    flush. During the day, my husband and I take 500–2,000 mg of
    inositol hexaniacinate without experiencing any side effects
    except the calm, even-headed feeling. Niacin is especially helpful
    after drinking caffeinated beverages to help calm the jitters. (I am
    not surprised to see it included in energy drinks that contain large
    amounts of stimulants.) You may also prefer to take flush-free
    niacin (inositol hexaniacinate) during the day for its calming
    effect and regular niacin at night. Before bed, the warm, flushing
    feeling of regular niacin relaxes the body and mind even further,
    but you avoid that sensation (and the rosy appearance) during the
    day by taking the flush-free variety.

11. You may find it interesting to learn more about the way your
    mind and body work and how to get on a natural schedule that

PAIN IN THE GUT: LYDIA'S STORY

Lydia was having digestive issues. She was also experiencing severe pain under her right rib, and anything she ate that had any sort of fat or oil would make the pain more excruciating. It was not uncommon for her to hover over the bathroom sink after meals, feeling like dinner was on its way back up. She ran her symptoms by her doc, and it seemed like there might be an issue with her gallbladder. Her grandmother had her gallbladder out. Maybe this was genetic. She went for an MRI, but nothing was found. No stones. No abnormalities. She appeared to be perfectly healthy. But her symptoms were persistent, real, and painful.

Lydia had been under a great deal of stress. Her acupuncturist, who was trying to help alleviate her migraines, told her that she had the "seven signs of stress." Along with her headaches, she was having trouble getting to sleep because she was overwhelmed with anxiety; she would get depressed and suffer mood swings; she was having sinus issues, fatigue, and concentration problems. And now, it hurt even to eat.

She knew she had to address the stress. She made a commitment to do just that and find ways to reduce her workload, integrate more exercise into her day, and decrease commitments, even when it was to do something fun. (Even good, happy stuff causes stress!) But it still hurt to eat *now,* and the doctors couldn't figure out why. She was hopeful things would get better over time with an attention to stress reduction, but she wanted something to help her symptoms right now.

She eventually found DoctorYourself.com and learned about the importance of a near-vegetarian diet rich in vitamin C and A, both protective of tissues. She read about the work of Garnett Cheney, M.D., and 100 of his patients, who healed their peptic ulcers by drinking a quart of raw cabbage juice every day. After a week, 81 percent of them were symptom-free. Dr. Cheney's cabbage juice protocol also had success with folks who had gastric ulcers and duodenal ulcers. He attributed it to what he called "Vitamin U" for lack of a better name.[81] She thought that if cabbage juice could heal painful, bleeding ulcers, maybe it could alleviate her gastrointestinal pain, too. She also felt safe, knowing she'd have a real hard time hurting herself with liquefied cabbage, although she was a bit chagrined about the whole idea as this wasn't exactly dignified dining. Cabbage juice sounded pretty unappetizing, but she was willing to do what it took to help heal her digestive pain.

She started juicing fresh, raw cabbage twice a day. She drank a pint glass full in the morning and another at dinnertime, along with her regular meals. She told me it tasted pretty awful (cabbage has kind of a spicy aftertaste that can be hard to get used to) but she'd plug her nose, chug it down, and chew on a piece of chocolate before letting go of her vice-grip on her nose, to be sure the aftertaste was only one of chocolate, not cabbage.

She didn't take a costly, glamorous drug; she didn't have to lie on an operating table. All she had to do was be brave enough to buy tons of inexpensive, bulk cabbage, be determined enough to ignore inquisitive stares from local grocers, and be dedicated enough to take the ten minutes twice a day to juice it and actually guzzle it down. Seven days later, her symptoms were gone, and they haven't returned since. She felt 100 percent better. It was totally worth it.

will promote good sleep.[72] One way to do this is to investigate Ayurveda, the time-honored folk medicine of India. To begin, you might want consider reading *Perfect Health* by Deepak Chopra and *Ayurveda: The Science of Self-Healing* by Vasant Lad.

12. Try eating a tablespoon or two of lecithin granules each day. Choline, found in lecithin as phosphatidylcholine, may help you stay asleep. Food sources of choline include milk, eggs, and peanuts.

Heart Disease and Stress

Stress wields its angry form in many ways, and one of the most serious consequences of long-term stress could be heart disease. This

SUPPLEMENT GUIDE FOR STRESS, ANXIETY, AND DEPRESSION

Vitamin A: 25,000 IU per day in the form of beta-carotene.

B-complex: Take one once or twice a day that contains 25–50 mg each of B_1, B_2, B_3, and B_6, and 400 mcg of folic acid; the amounts of B_{12}, biotin, and pantothenic acid can vary.

Vitamin B$_3$: When needed, take an additional 50–500 mg of nicotinic acid, or try 500–1,000 mg "flush-free" (inositol hexaniacinate) niacin, or take 100–500 mg of niacinamide. Note that these are "as needed" amounts, so your total daily dose may be higher or lower depending on your symptoms.

Calcium: In the form of carbonate or citrate, take 1,000–2,000 mg per day; take separately from your iron supplement.

Chromium: In the form of chromium picolinate, take 200–400 mcg a day. For depression, take up to1,000 mcg per day.

Vitamin C: 6,000–18,000 mg per day; take more or less as needed.

Vitamin E: 400 IU per day in the form of mixed tocopherols or d-alpha tocopherol; take separately from your iron supplement.

Vitamin D: 1,000–2,000 IU per day.

Iron: In the form of ferrous fumarate, ferrous gluconate, or carbonyl iron, take 18 mg per day; take separately from your vitamin E and calcium supplements.

Magnesium: In the form of citrate or gluconate, take 400–1,000 mg per day or more as needed.

Omega-3 fatty acids: Look for a fish oil supplement that contains 900–1,000 mg total of EPA and DHA omega-3 fatty acids. A tablet that contains 1,000 mg of fish oil may only contain 300 mg of omega-3 fatty acids. You will want to take three of those a day to get the optimum dose.

Selenium: 100–200 mcg a day.

Multivitamin: Take twice daily. Look for one that contains 15–30 mg of zinc, too.

Inositol: For anxiety and related disorders, take 500 mg-18 grams daily.

Lecithin: Take in the form of granules; one tablespoon daily.

is *very* serious stuff. According to the American Heart Association, cardiovascular disease is the leading killer of women.[73] "Nearly twice as many women in the United States die of heart disease, stroke, and other cardiovascular diseases as from all forms of cancer, including breast cancer."[74] "Among all U.S. women who die each year, one in four dies of heart disease. In 2004, nearly 60 percent more women died of cardiovascular disease (heart disease and stroke) than from all cancers combined."[75]

Much contributes to our risk for heart disease including diabetes, high blood pressure, too much bad LDL cholesterol and not enough good HDL cholesterol, being overweight, being a smoker, and that it might run in our family. Stress can also be a factor behind heart disease because so many things we do or have as a result of stress add to our risk factors. For example, stress may encourage overeating and weight gain, which also contributes to a higher risk for diabetes; stress might keep us from not getting enough exercise; it can raise our blood pressure; it can raise our cholesterol levels when we eat a poorly; it could contribute to our smoking habit. For this reason, doing what we can to minimize our stress level and the associated stress-induced behaviors and health risks is critically important—and so is taking our vitamins.

A study of over 87,000 women found that those who took at least 100 IU of vitamin E each day for two years reduced their risk of heart disease by over half.[76] Even relatively small amounts of supplemental vitamin C can help save lives. One study of over 85,000 women showed that vitamin C supplementation reduced the risk of coronary heart disease.[77] Niacin (nicotinic acid) is extremely effective at building up that good cholesterol in our body and reducing the bad,[78] which is exactly what we need to decrease our risk of heart disease. It has been referred to as the "most effective medication in current clinical use for increasing high-density lipoprotein (HDL) cholesterol."[79] In fact, it's *more* effective at raising good cholesterol HDL levels than those prescription meds we see advertised on TV all the time, and niacin is far cheaper and far safer, too.[80]

Stiff, Achy, and Painful Joints

Do you have aches, pain, and stiffness in your joints? Do you have trouble bending your knees or grasping with your hands? Stress can contribute to such aches and pains. You may want to start supplementing with niacinamide. William Kaufman, M.D., successfully treated joint dysfunction with niacinamide with anywhere from 400 to 2,250 mg per day in divided doses.[82] You could start with 100 mg at each meal, and then increase your dose until you experience relief just like Kaufman's patients did.

THE DIFFICULT PART

When you are depressed, anxious, or just completely stressed out, sometimes it feels like it will be this way forever. It's hard to cope with the moment, let alone the idea that you have the next hour, day, week, month, or year to face. But right now, you can begin to take control.

Stress is a part of life, but it can be managed without drugs. Proactively organize your day in such a way that you reduce stressors, and incorporate coping strategies for the stress you can't eliminate.

Anxiety and depression can be very serious conditions, and it's no wonder that so many folks will turn to medication hoping for some relief. Arguably, there are people out there who truly need drugs to manage their mind, but perhaps you will be able to effectively manage yours with nutrition. You can always choose to take pharmaceuticals, but it does no harm to try nutrition first. Don't fool yourself into thinking it is "easier" to just take a drug. Side effects can have quite a negative impact, if you don't know that already. If the mood extremes of anxiety and depression are your "normal," know that it doesn't have to be that way. Take the steps necessary to give your body a fighting chance with proper nutrition, vitamins, minerals, and lifestyle adjustments.

As my father always says, "Life is not one mood long." It is annoying to hear (and perhaps for you to read) especially if you are currently feel in crisis, but it rings true, mostly in retrospect. Whether you are panicked and feel like you are losing it, or just so depressed you can't face the world, the hardest thing to do may be to stop yourself, acknowledge that your feelings are real, and then take just one healthy step to improve the moment. That's the hard part. There is a whole life ahead of you that can be better, and that's worth working for.

RECOMMENDED READING

Challem, J. *The Food Mood Solution*. Hoboken, NJ: John Wiley & Sons, 2007.

Hoffer, A., A. W. Saul. *Orthomolecular Medicine for Everyone: Megavitamin Therapeutics for Families and Physicians*. Laguna Beach, CA: Basic Health Publications, 2008.

Hoffer A., A. W. Saul, H. D. Foster. *Niacin: The Real Story*. Laguna Beach, CA: Basic Health Publications, 2011.

Hoffer, A., J. Prousky. *Anxiety: Orthomolecular Diagnosis and Treatment*. Toronto, ON: CCNM Press, 2006.

Kaufman, W. *The Common Form of Joint Dysfunction*. Brattleboro, VT: E.L. Hildreth and Co., 1949. Full text available online at: http://www.DoctorYourself.com/ kaufman6.html. (accessed October 2011).

Levy, T. E. *Stop America's #1 Killer: Reversible Vitamin Deficiency Found to Be Origin of ALL Coronary Heart Disease*. Henderson, NV: Livon Books, 2006.

Pauling, L. *How to Live Longer and Feel Better*. Corvallis, OR: Oregon State University Press, 2006.

Prousky, J. *The Vitamin Cure for Chronic Fatigue Syndrome*. Laguna, Beach, CA: Basic Health Publications, 2010.

CHAPTER 6

PROBLEMS WITH THE PILL AND OTHER FORMS OF HORMONAL BIRTH CONTROL

"I want to tell you a terrific story
about oral contraception.
I asked this girl to sleep with me
and she said 'No.' "
—WOODY ALLEN

Hormonal birth control advertisements make their products seem quite alluring: their commercials and websites are filled with pastel colors, images of flowers, trendy designs, and beautiful, independent women donning huge smiles. There are obvious reasons why these drugs are so appealing; we hardly need sappy commercials to suggest them to us. We are looking for a simple, spontaneous, clean, and convenient way to have sex without worrying about making a baby. We want some control over what happens to our bodies; we want to be able to decide when (and if) we get pregnant.

Sometimes, we may even consider using hormonal birth control for something other than pregnancy prevention. Did your doctor recommend (advertise) the ring, patch, pill, or implant to you? No more cramps![1] Regulate your period! Get rid of acne![2] Help alleviate pain from endometriosis![3] Premenstrual syndrome (PMS) symptoms will improve! Reduce your risk for endometrial cancer and ovarian cancer![4] While some women may find relief when using hormonal birth control, other women find they just trade one discomfort for another.

The Pill for Reasons Other than Pregnancy Prevention

Hormonal contraceptives are prescribed for numerous reasons other than their obvious purpose. Many symptoms we are attempting to alleviate, such as cramps or premenstrual syndrome (PMS) symptoms, can also be managed with nutrition, exercise, vitamins, and an overall healthy lifestyle. Check out other chapters in this book for helpful suggestions.

It seems, at least in my experience, that my doctors spent more time "selling" these prescriptions to me than they did reviewing all of the potential side effects. Perhaps I was too young to fully appreciate what I was getting myself into, but how many other young women aren't getting all the information they need to make a fully informed decision? In fairness, maybe we just aren't listening. Perhaps we are too busy thinking only of the benefits of using hormonal contraceptives and not the negative consequences of adding drugs to our system.

The trouble with hormonal birth control is that when you use it, little besides child prevention is truly under our control. Depression? Severe headaches? Painful sex? Anxiety? Recurrent yeast and bacterial vaginosis? Difficulty sleeping? Outright craziness? Cramps? Do any of these problems sound familiar to you?

THE SIDE EFFECTS

You don't have to go far to find out what kind of side effects can be caused by your hormonal birth control. Next time you pick up your prescription, pause before you throw out all of that written material. Start reading that tissue-thin insert that comes with every purchase.

If you can't wait until next month's visit to the pharmacy, I've got you covered. Here are the side effects associated with the use of the pill, at least the ones the drug companies admit to.

You have an increased risk of experiencing the following if you use oral contraceptives: thrombophlebitis (a blot clot that forms deep in your body), arterial thromboembolism (a blood clot in an artery), pulmonary embolism (a blood clot in the lung), myocardial infarction (heart attack), cerebral hemorrhage (stroke), cerebral thrombosis (a blood clot that prevents blood from getting to the brain), hypertension (high blood pressure), gallbladder disease, and hepatic adenomas (liver tumors that can become malignant, hemorrhage, or rupture) or benign liver tumors.[8]

Maybe they should just write: the pill might kill you.

Other side effects associated with hormonal contraceptive use include: nausea; vomiting; gastrointestinal symptoms (such as abdominal cramps and bloating); breakthrough bleeding; spotting; change in menstrual flow; amenorrhea (menstruation stops); temporary infertility after discontinuation of treatment; edema (accumulation of fluid behind the skin); melasma (darkening or discoloration of the skin); breast changes such as tenderness, enlargement, and/or secretion; change in weight (increase or decrease); change in cervical erosion and secretion (discharge differences); reduction in lactation when

THE POPULAR PILL

Who is taking the pill? A whole bunch of us. In the United States, the birth control pill is the most commonly used form of contraception for women between the ages of fifteen and twenty-nine.[5] After the age of twenty-nine, when women start deciding to stop having children, sterilization becomes the preferred method of preventing pregnancy, but the pill still remains the second-most popular choice of birth control.[6] As you might expect, young women in these age groups are also most likely to be the ones having children, as 85 percent of births occur in women under the age of thirty-five.[7] This means that for women in the child bearing years between the ages fifteen and thirty-four, the pill is the preferred choice of birth control *over any other method*. That's a lot of ladies on drugs.

SUBTLE SIDE EFFECTS OF THE PILL: SELECTING OUR SWEETHEART

Not all of the side effects of the pill are obvious. Evidence is emerging that shows that taking the birth control pill may alter male and female mate choice. Here's the scoop: when we are fertile (not on the pill), we subconsciously prefer the smell of men that have a dissimilar MHC genotype (a group of genes that play an important role in immune function), a selection process that may increase genetic diversity in our kids and reduce inbreeding, both of which are evolutionarily preferable.[10] Taking oral contraceptives messes with all of that. Pill users are more likely to prefer the smell of MHC *similar* men.[11] It is believed this occurs because the body is fooled into thinking that the pill user is pregnant, and evolutionarily, it is important to have family members around to protect us during this time. In other words, the pill changes what odors we find alluring.

Additionally, men also happen to find us most attractive when we are mid-cycle and most likely to be fertile.[12] Our odor changes throughout our natural menstrual cycle, and men seem to be able to identify ovulation based on our smell.[13] But when we are on the pill, our natural hormones, and our odors, are distorted in such a way that it affects a man's natural cyclical preferences.[14] Taking the pill doesn't seem to change whether or not they find us attractive, but their interest no longer correlates with our menstrual cycle.[15] Why does this matter? Well, if our (or our man's) selection process is skewed, we may be getting involved in a relationship that is less likely to succeed. Since pairing with an "evolutionarily preferred" dissimilar mate may ultimately affect our contentment with a relationship and its resilience and our reproductive outcomes, we have to ask ourselves whether the pill is affecting one of the most significant decisions we ever make: whom we want to be with.[16]

given immediately postpartum; cholestatic jaundice (yellowing due to changes in bile flow); migraine; allergic reactions including rash, urticaria (hives), and/or angioedema (swelling beneath the skin); mental depression; reduced tolerance to carbohydrates; vaginal candidiasis (yeast infections); steepening of corneal curvature (bulging of the cornea, which can cause scarring that can impair vision); and intolerance to contact lenses.[9] Or, to make a long story short, the pill might make you absolutely miserable.

This is not even a complete list. It's more of an overview of the common ailments associated with oral contraceptives. There are also many other patient-reported side effects associated with pill use that have not been "confirmed or denied." That's a nice way of saying, "Sorry ladies, we don't believe you."

Oh, but what about the patch, the ring, or the implant? They are better, right? If you think using hormonal birth control other than the pill reduces your risk of side effects, you are mistaken. The generous list of side effects for the ring, patch, and implant won't comfort you any.

Once you start experiencing the symptoms of a serious condition caused by hormonal contraceptive use, *it means you already have a problem.* Even more serious complications, like dying, can result, and that is no way to find out that taking the pill wasn't a good idea.

Is this meant to startle you? You bet. Too many of us quietly, punctually, and without question, use these medications without being fully aware of the possible consequences.

Clara's Story

For some women I have spoken to about the pill, it didn't necessarily start out all bad, but it sure ended that way. Sometimes it takes a while to discover what is really at the center of your illnesses, and for Clara, it took a decade.

As a college student with no desire to get pregnant in the near future and content with her monogamous long-term relationship with her boyfriend, Clara decided it would be a great option to go on the pill. She looked forward to the convenience and reliability of

"IT'S YOUR VAGINA THAT'S THE PROBLEM."

Sue said:

"My doctor actually spoke those words to me. After hearing my complaints about how badly I was feeling when I switched to the vaginal contraceptive ring, my doctor informed me that it wasn't the drug, but my vagina that was the problem. Oh. What I was experiencing couldn't possibly be due to the ring, he said. It must be me.

My vagina is just fine, thank you. The ring was the issue, and I knew it. I went home, I removed it, I felt better, and I fired my doctor."

It's scary to go against what your doctor says. It's easy to second-guess yourself and believe they are right; after all, they have the medical degree.

This is where it gets tough. You know how you feel. You know how you should feel. You are very good at noticing changes within your body; you need to trust yourself and what you are experiencing.

Don't let someone try to convince you that your symptoms are "just you" and have nothing to do with the contraceptive drugs you are using. If there is any question, rule out the possibility that the drug is the issue. The only way to do that is to stop taking it, and see if you feel better.

regulated periods. She and her boyfriend had also tested negative for sexually transmitted diseases, so the pill, like for so many women, seemed the preferred method of birth control.

At first, the pill's side effects were tolerable. For the first few years, Clara noticed stronger mood swings, ranging from pure bliss to downright depression. She attributed this to being a highly emotional college student under what she considered to be a great deal of stress.

Then she returned home and switched brands. It was cheaper to get something different, and her gynecologist said it would be okay. But things were not okay. Clara became more and more affected by side effects. Each pill that she switched to, to get rid of the problems the last one was causing, just ended up giving her a whole new set of problems to worry about. And they were usually more expensive, too.

Here came the dilemma: she, like so many women on the pill, enjoyed the spontaneity other birth control methods couldn't provide. She wasn't ready to give up on the obvious benefits of taking an oral contraceptive, even if she had to deal with some side effects. So, instead of going off the pill, she began to chart the side effects to find out which drug would work best for her.

Clara charted a full year of migraine headaches, some that would occur each day for two and sometimes for up to three weeks of every month, that were so bad an MRI was ordered to check to see if she had a brain tumor. Her doctors never told her the pill could be to blame, but she suspected otherwise.

She switched a few more times, even went back to the pill she orginally started taking (see table on following page), and finally got rid of those headaches, but now she was getting yeast infections every month to every other month. This wasn't even on her chart. It hadn't occurred to her that this was a direct result of taking the pill, and her doctor never suggested the idea either. Neither she nor her doctor had put two and two together, so for about three years she "managed" each outbreak of infection with medicine, assuming this was just "her."

On her own, Clara read about ways to control yeast. She changed everything in her life to battle the invaders. She put herself on a very bland no-sugar, no-alcohol diet. She started taking medication regularly, not just during an outbreak, to fight and to prevent infection. She took herbs and ate yogurt every day. No matter how drastically she tried to combat the yeast, nothing fixed the problem.

After *four years* of infection after infection, she finally got to thinking that it must be due to the pill. Nothing else could account for it. If having recurrent vaginal infections doesn't destroy spontaneity and intimacy, what does? She decided that maybe she shouldn't be taking oral birth control at all.

CLARA'S PILL SYMPTOMS CHART

	ORTHO TRI-CYCLEN	DESOGEN	APRI	KARIVA	NUVA-RING	PATCH	ORTHO TRI-CYCLEN
Bad Mood Swings	Yes	Some	Yes	Yes	Yes		Yes
Migraine Headaches	No	No	Yes	Some	Yes		Yes
Lowered Sex Drive	No	No	No	No	Yes		No
Spotting	No	No	No	Yes	No		No
Nausea	Some	Some	Yes	Yes	Yes		Some
Depression	Some	Some	No	No	Yes		Some
Cramps/Pain	No	No	Yes	Yes	Yes		No
Yeast Infections	No	No	No	Yes	Yes		Yes
Painful Sex	No	No	No	No	Yes		Yes
Negative Testimony from Other Users	Little	Little	A lot	Some	A lot	Lawsuits! I won't use it.	Little
Cost	$$$	$$	$	$	$$$	$$$	$$$

After a total of ten years of being a guinea pig, she took a huge step: she went off the pill and chose an alternative nonhormonal method of birth control. Her doctors were still convinced that the drug wasn't at the root of the problem, but Clara had had enough. She didn't experience some of the really serious adverse consequences some suffer from due to the pill: she didn't get cancer (at least not yet), she didn't have a heart attack, stroke, or venous thrombo-embolism (the formation of blood clots, also known as VTE). For her, the symptoms she was experiencing were life-damaging enough.

Since she stopped taking the pill, Clara hasn't had a migraine headache. Her mood swings are normal, manageable events that she can effectively control with vitamin therapy. Sex is no longer painful or uncomfortable, and her sex drive has returned to where it should be. Cramps are minimal to none and can be managed with vitamin therapy. Her minor anxiety and depression, familiar to most menstruating women who experience some level of PMS, can also be managed with good health. Most importantly, she no longer is getting recurrent yeast infections. Now she can actually have sex.

Cancer of the Breast, Cervix, and Liver

Not all of the side effects of oral contraceptives are listed in the packaging. I guess putting the warning *"May cause cancer"* on the label might reduce profits. Of course, cigarette companies have managed just fine.

When you take oral contraceptives, you significantly increase your chances of getting breast cancer.[17] Your risk of breast cancer is higher if you take the pill and are under the age of thirty-five,[18] the same gals that just so happen to be the most likely group to use this form of birth control. The risk for breast cancer continues to increase if you have been on the pill for more than ten years.[19] The risk is even higher if you began using the pill as a teenager.[20] Interestingly, after you stop using the pill (and have ceased to use it for ten years), your risk of breast cancer goes down and becomes no greater than that of non-pill users.[21] In other words, the pill is safe, as long as you don't take it anymore.

Use oral contraceptives for over five years, and you increase your risk of cervical cancer.[22] The human papillomavirus (HPV) is considered to be the main culprit of cervical cancer, but evidence shows that if you have HPV and you are on the pill for over five years, you are up to *four times* more likely to get cervical cancer than a non-pill user.[23] You are *three times* more likely than non-users to get cervical cancer if you have HPV and began taking the pill before the age of twenty.[24] And, if you have taken the pill within the last five years, your risk for cervical cancer is also increased.[25] After cessation of the pill, data suggest that your risk for cervical cancer decreases,[26] another good reason to quit taking it.

And, to top it all off, your risk for liver cancer also significantly increases if you take oral contraceptives.[27] Oh, goodie.

How Common Are Serious Side Effects?

If I was told that taking a pill would significantly increase my chances of getting killed in a motor vehicle accident, I would think twice before swallowing. I know too many people that have perished on the road, and I really don't want to be one of them.

If you take oral contraceptives, you can double and even triple your chances of having a heart attack, stroke, VTE, and, for women under the age of thirty-five, breast cancer.[28] Your chances multiply if you smoke, are obese, have high blood pressure, or have diabetes.[29] However, it can be argued (and from the studies I have read it often is) that even doubled or tripled, the risk of having any one of these problems is still small. For example, if you take oral contraceptives, your estimated yearly risk of acquiring VTE is less than 3 in 10,000; you have about a 3 in one million chance of heart attack; and you have about a 22 in 100,000 chance of having a stroke.[30] But if you do a little rough math and add those numbers up with a common denominator, each year women on the pill have approximately a 50 in 100,000 combined risk of experiencing one of these serious ailments.

Hold that thought; now let's talk cancer. It has been estimated that for every 100,000 women who *do not* use the pill, 2,782 will develop breast cancer, 425 will develop cervical cancer, and 20 with get liver cancer. If oral contraceptives have been used for eight years, it is estimated that an additional 151 women will get breast cancer, an additional 125 women will be diagnosed with cancer of the cervix, and additional 41 women will get liver cancer.[31] This means that about 317 more women per 100,000 will get cancer if they have been on oral contraceptives. Add that number up with the yearly risk of stroke, heart attack, and VTE, and we have an estimated additional 367 cases per 100,000 of significant, serious side effects experienced by women who use oral contraceptives.

In 2002, approximately 11.6 million women were using the pill as their contraception method.[32] If you take that figure of 367 per

100,000 and multiply that out, approximately 42,572 women who were taking the pill in 2002 are now, in 2010, going to experience serious, adverse consequences due to their eight years of pill use. That's 42,572 cases of preventable disease. Perhaps that number seems small compared to the 11 million women who won't have these problems. Or, perhaps it's just not a big deal, as long as one of those 42,572 women isn't you or someone you love.

Some medical literature attempts to convince us of the low "attributable risk" of contraceptive pill consumption. Because so few women get, say, liver cancer, even a doubling or tripling of their risk due to oral contraceptives still means only a relatively small number will be affected. It is argued that your risk is not significant. One article suggests, for example, that the risks associated with oral contraceptive use can be compared favorably with the risks of common events like, for example, car accidents.[33] According to the National Safety Council, each year we have about a 15 in 100,000 chance of dying in a motor vehicle accident.[34] So, with a possible 367 per 100,000 women experiencing just some of the serious pill-related side effects, we are about twenty-four times *more* likely to suffer from a serious complication due to oral contraceptive use than we are likely to die in a car accident going to the pharmacy to get them.

Well, that doesn't calm me down one bit. How about you?

LOW-DOSE PILLS AND OTHER FORMS OF HORMONAL CONTRACEPTION

So what's with the creation of all these new low-dose preparations? The short answer is that people were dying. We have low-dose pills now because studies show that the pills of yesteryear had way too high a concentration of hormones. Incidences of thromboembolic events (like heart attacks and stroke) are directly related to the dose of estrogen[35] in the pill, and therefore the major reason why low-dose pills were created was to "reduce the incidence of adverse cardiovascular side effects."[36] In the 1960s, oral contraceptives contained 150 mcg of synthetic estrogen, whereas most pills prescribed today have 35 mcg or less.[37] For example, one study demonstrated a 60 percent decrease in deaths from cardiovascular events when estrogen (ethinyl estradiol) doses were decreased from 50 to 35 mcg.[38] Even lower-dose pills are out now, with only 20 mcg of estrogen.

Does "low-dose" mean safer? Maybe the better question is: do you feel like finding out? Current class-action lawsuits against some popular low-dose pills draw attention to the fact that people are still dying. So, no. Low-dose pills are not necessarily safer.

There are so many different forms of the pill out there. New hormone preparations, combinations, and concentrations keep working their way into the market. We spend, at best, an average of fifteen to twenty minutes with our doctors when we visit them; just how much information do they really find out about us, or have time to give to us, when it comes to selecting the right pill? In their defense, doctors can't be fully aware of all potential issues for all potential users because in many cases, especially with newer drugs, those issues are yet to be discovered.

Consider this: It's hard to find long-term clinical studies about the ring, the patch, and the newer forms of hormonal contraceptives. That's because in many cases, they're waiting for us to try them out and see what happens. And considering that drug companies are hesitant to test their own products thoroughly because they might look bad,[39] it means that the only way we know if they are truly harmful is to test the products for them, and pay for the privilege.

Sometimes the next "new thing" captures our attention, and we want to try it. But ladies, we aren't talking about getting the latest fashion in footwear. As fabulous and as easy as advertisements make hormonal contraceptives out to be, for many of us there is a price to pay with our health. Will we be fortunate and breeze on by without side effects? Or, will we end up being one of the women who help drive up statistics and motivate scientists to go back to the laboratory?

We shouldn't claim that we didn't know any better. There are numerous studies that show the consequences of using hormonal contraceptives. There are numerous lawsuits showcasing the harm they can cause. There are many women who are suffering and dying, and more will follow. Yet, there are millions of us still using the drugs.

BE INFORMED

Go read the side effects section of your birth control pill drug facts insert. Lost it? Grab the *Physician's Desk Reference* from your local library (unless you want to pony up the seventy bucks to buy the latest edition) or just go online to www.pdr.net or one of the other drug information websites like www.rxlist.com or www.drugs.com, which put all this knowledge right at your fingertips for free. These resources will give you more details than the folks at the pharmacy will. Once you have the information at hand, don't take anything listed lightly. Know what you are getting yourself into. Pay attention to your body and how you feel; that awareness will help you decide what is best for you.

I guess you have to ask yourself just one question: do you feel lucky?

Well, do ya?

IF YOU INSIST ON TAKING THE PILL, TAKE YOUR VITAMINS TOO

We can't pretend that taking hormonal contraceptives is without risk, and I'm not suggesting that vitamins eliminate your chances of experiencing side effects, serious or otherwise. However, if you are going to use hormonal contraceptives, you should be aware that your need for certain vitamins increases.

Doctors have known for over four decades that vitamins and hormonal birth control use should go hand in hand. Serum levels of vitamin B_2 (riboflavin), vitamin B_6 (pyridoxine), vitamin C, folic acid, and vitamin B_{12} levels may be reduced when we take the pill.[40] Additionally, the metabolism of the pill by our liver requires extra amounts of certain nutrients: B-complex, vitamin C, magnesium, and zinc.[41] Furthermore, the pill interferes with the absorption of folic acid, vitamin B_6, selenium, and vitamin C, which just makes it harder to avoid shortages. Therefore, if you are taking the pill and you are not taking more of the vitamins and minerals your body requires, you could be generating deficiencies.

Deficiencies of vitamin B_6 cause depression, irritability, and serious issues like atherosclerosis, which can lead to heart attack and stroke; lack of folic acid leads to fatigue, headaches, and more serious issues like anemia; B_{12} deficiency can lead to such symptoms as fatigue, depression, and irritability; vitamin C deficiency weakens your immune system; and deficiency of the mineral magnesium can cause cramping and fatigue. Look carefully at this abbreviated list of just *some* of the symptoms experienced by the vitamin deficient individual. Notice any similarities between this list and the list of side effects on your pack of oral contraceptives?

The B Vitamins

It makes sense to B-sure you are taking enough of the Bs, especially if you are taking hormonal birth control.

For example, women on the pill have significantly reduced levels of B_6 and B_{12}.[42] So let's connect some dots. We know, and have known for some time, that a deficiency of B_6 can cause hardening of the arteries (atherosclerosis), a condition that can lead to heart attack and stroke.[43] You can't ignore that taking the pill increases your risk for heart attack and stroke. Could this be due to vitamin deficiency? Low levels of B_6 are also associated with an increased risk for blot clots,[44] another possible side effect of pill use. It has also been found that higher levels of folate (B_9, aka folic acid) and B_6 may reduce the risk of breast cancer[45] as do higher levels of B_{12} and folate,[46] the same vitamins found to be deficient in pill users, who also happen to be at greater risk for breast cancer. If women on the pill have reduced levels of B vitamins, and deficiencies can cause serious disease (that are also attributed to pill use), doesn't it make sense that pill users should take more of the Bs?

How do you do that? The best way, as always, is through your food. Fruits and green leafy veggies are the best sources of B_6 and B_{12}. Citrus fruits, tomatoes, vegetables, and grain products are good sources of folic acid.[47] You can obtain the United States Recommeded Dietary Allowance (RDA) of B_6 (2 mg or even less depending on age), B_{12} (about 2.5 mcg), and folic acid (400 mcg) with a very health-conscious diet, but these small levels are difficult to obtain even if you are paying close attention to what you eat every single day, and you may find it quite impossible to provide yourself with therapeutic levels of B vitamins. Studies showed that taking B_6 (240–250 mg) and folic acid (5–10 mg) each day was associated with a decreased risk of atherosclerosis, with *no side effects*.[48] To get the 250 mg of B_6 shown to help reduce your chance of atherosclerosis, you would need to eat about 360 bananas a day or 890 cups of cooked spinach.[49] Hopefully you don't have much else to do today! Sure, you should eat plenty of spinach and bananas, but supplementation is a far more expedient way of getting the vitamins you need without excessive eating!

Supplementation is necessary if your need is greater. If you are on the pill, or have taken the pill in the past, *your need is greater*. In fact, one study showed that 75 percent of women who use oral contraceptives and do not take B_6 supplements are deficient in B_6.[50] Even among women who no longer take the pill, 40 percent were found to

HOMOCYSTEINE: WHAT IS IT AND WHY SHOULD WE CARE?

Homocysteine is an amino acid in blood. High levels of homocysteine are caused by deficiencies in certain nutrients, namely B vitamins and magnesium, and it contributes to an increased risk for heart disease, stroke, and atherosclerosis.[53] Folic acid,[54] other B vitamins such as B_6 and B_{12},[55] and magnesium[56] help break down homocysteine, and in adequate amounts, they help reduce the likelihood that you'll get atherosclerosis or even more serious conditions like stroke and heart disease. Since these diseases are all risk factors for women on the pill, it makes sense to compensate for deficiencies by eating a healthy diet and taking supplements.

still be deficient in B_6.[51] Another noteworthy comparison: former users of oral contraceptives were also found to have significantly higher levels of homocysteine than never-users.[52]

Feeling cranky lately? If you are trying to manage mood swings, you may need more B vitamins. The pill can increase the severity of these mood swings, and therefore, your need for the Bs may go up. Mood swings happen to be one of the most easily recognizable symptoms of B-vitamin deficiency, so it's a good place to start if you are wondering whether or not you need supplements. Taking birth control can make you feel more depressed, especially when you are already prone to depression. Taking B_6 may help prevent and alleviate symptoms of depression while you are taking the pill.[57] But how much do you take? Good question. The Bs work best when taken together, so if you are taking the pill, start with a good B-complex at least once a day. Find a tablet that gives you 50 mg each of B_1, B_2, B_3 (niacinamide), and B_6, keeping in mind that you may need to take more B_6.[58] B_6 is particularly effective in dealing with irritability, anxiety, tension, depression, and PMS mood changes because it works with folate, B_{12}, and tryptophan to make serotonin, that feel-good neurotransmitter.[59] As a general rule, you may want to take another 50–100 mg per day of B_6 along with your B-complex. For an acute episode, also known as "I'm-going-to-throw-a-chair-through-a-window," take 100–200 mg of B_6 and your B-complex right then and there. You may find yourself being able to put that chair down in about half an hour.

B Vitamin Safety

Experiencing side effects from B vitamins is rare, but with anything, it is prudent to know what could happen if you took way too much, even if your chances of experiencing any side effects are small. For example, very high doses (2,000–6,000 mg per day) of B_6, specifically, taken *by itself* without the other complementary B vitamins, may cause neurological symptoms such as temporary tingling, nervousness, and numbness, which will cease once supplementation stops.[60] Adding one to two *hundred* milligrams of B_6 to your daily diet, not *thousands* of milligrams, means it is unlikely you will experience any side effects from your dosage of supplemental B_6, especially when taken along with a B-complex vitamin.[61]

No known dose of B_1, B_2, or B_{12} is toxic.[62] If you are taking a B-complex once or twice a day that contains 50 mg of B_1, 50 mg of B_2, and 50 mcg of B_{12}, you should "B" all set. Most people find these amounts to be well-tolerated.

The recommended daily amount of folic acid is 400 mcg a day and 600 mcg if you are pregnant; both amounts happen to be difficult to obtain from food sources alone even if you are paying close attention to your diet. Your B-complex is likely to contain 400 mcg folic acid, and even if you take two of those a day and get some more in a good multivitamin, you are not overdoing it. Not to worry, folic acid is not toxic.[63]

You can't kill yourself with B_3 either. B_3 comes in several forms, and which one you take depends on what you prefer. A B-complex containing 50 mg of niacinamide or inositol hexaniacinate, taken once or twice daily, is a good start. Regular niacin, in the form of nicotinic acid, may make you feel itchy and "flushed" like when you have a sun burn. Some folks prefer to stay away from this form of niacin because they find the side effects, though completely harmless, unnerving.[64] My husband and I prefer to take a small amount (50–200 mg or even more if we're super stressed) of regular niacin before bed, as it calms us and the warming sensation helps us fall asleep, especially if we have thoughts spinning through our heads. I've never had to take a sleep aid (although I've wanted to) because I take niacin instead. My husband used to have difficulty falling asleep, but not since he's met me. B_3 is even more easily tolerated when it is taken with vitamin C or on a full stomach. You may find, over time, that you stop flushing if you take nicotinic acid regularly. Even in extremely high doses, like the 5,000 to 30,000 mg used to treat patients with schizophrenia, niacin is shown to be nontoxic.[65] B_3 is good to take if you are feeling especially anxious, nervous, twitchy, irritable, or moody. Take an extra 100–500 mg of niacinamide or 50–200 mg of nicotinic acid or 500–1,000 of flush-free niacin (inositol hexaniacinate) to manage those acute episodes.

WHY CAN'T YOU TELL ME EXACTLY HOW MUCH I NEED TO TAKE?

We often get nervous when we aren't given exact dosages. I don't blame you for feeling that way, especially if you are learning about vitamins for the first time. We are so used to taking pharmaceuticals that are universally measured out in such a way that practically everyone gets the same amount of medicine. Vitamins work differently. Think about this: the amount of a pharmaceutical drug an adult takes may differ from that of a child, but adults vary a lot, don't they? Gender, size, diet, lifestyle, culture . . . it goes on. I really don't find it odd that you have to adjust your intake of vitamins based on your need. I find it far weirder that drugs are given out in so many standardized dosages. But that's because they're *dangerous.* Not so with vitamins. To find how much of a vitamin you need, you simply have to take it and pay attention to how you feel, even if it ends up being a lot. Have your symptoms improved? Are they unchanged? Are you experiencing any side effects? You may need to take more; you may need to take less. You have to be willing to trust yourself to take care of yourself. The best part is: vitamins are so *safe.* Even if you think you've "screwed up" and perhaps taken too much, it is extremely unlikely that you will kill yourself. According to the recent American Association of Poison Control Centers' 27th annual report, *nobody* died from taking vitamins.[66] Nobody! The same cannot be said about drugs. You have a great deal more flexibility to monitor and adjust your vitamin intake, whereas you can't (and shouldn't) do this with pharmaceutical drugs.

Vitamin C

Vitamin C is going to end up in every chapter in this book, and this is why: it is absolutely essential. It also happens to be very safe and virtually nontoxic.[67] You'll be surprised at how taking even a small dose (2,000 mg) will make you feel so much *better.* Now, I realize that "small" amount may not seem so little to you. Heck, the RDA is only about 75 mg per day. Isn't 2,000 mg a bit excessive? If we eat just a couple of small packages of Skittles we've got the RDA covered! Before you run off and start popping these candy-coated confections, I'm *not* even remotely suggesting that you obtain your vitamin C from artificially colored, artificially flavored, sugar-laden snacks. What I am suggesting is that the RDA is way too low, and that we should be appalled that a king-size bag of Skittles may indeed be someone's idea of an adequate way to get their daily vitamin C. Therapeutic levels of vitamin C happen to be *much* higher than the level determined by the RDA. Scientist Linus Pauling, who won not one but *two* unshared Nobel Prizes (which no one else in history has done), is in the minds of many, the definitive source on the topic of vitamin C. He recommends that you take anywhere from 6,000–18,000 mg a day, an amount quite impossible to obtain through diet alone.[68] To know how much vitamin C you personally should take, note how much it takes to reach bowel tolerance (diarrhea); at that point, you know you have taken too much. This is a harmless side effect, but it can be inconvenient, so make sure you can test your limits on a day when you don't have to, say, sit quietly at your kid's violin recital. The amount just below bowel tolerance is the amount of C to take regularly, and this will vary for each individual. The more C you need because of stress, oral contraceptives, sickness, etc., the more you can tolerate. Be sure to divide your dose: for example, take 2,000 mg in the morning, 2,000 mg at lunch, and another 2,000 mg at dinnertime. Taking vitamin C while you are on the pill (and even if you aren't) will help boost your immune system so will be less likely to get infections. It will also help elevate your mood and increase your overall energy level.

MINERALS

Add magnesium (500–1,000 mg) to your supplement list if you are on the pill (and even if you aren't). Nearly 70 percent of us aren't even getting the recommended daily amounts of magnesium, let alone optimal levels.[69] If you are one of the many women who have to cope with menstrual cramps, read more about how magnesium can "Curtail Your Cramps" in Chapter 2.

Zinc is another nutrient we may not get enough of. The RDA is not at all high: a mere 8–13 mg per day is recommended for us gals.[70] If you happen to be over the age of sixty, it is likely that you aren't even getting the low recommended dosage of zinc.[71] Take at least 15 mg per day,[72] but two or three times this amount is still very safe.

THE PILLS YOU NEED TO TAKE WITH "THE PILL"

If you are taking hormonal birth control, it is likely that you need more of the following nutrients. Divide your doses and take with meals.

B-complex: Take one twice a day that contains 25–50 mg each of B_1, B_2, B_3, and B_6, 25–50 mcg of B_{12}, and 400 mcg of folic acid.

Vitamin B_3: When needed, take an additional 50–500 mg per day of nicotinic acid; or try 500–1,000 mg per day of "flush-free" (inositol hexaniacinate) niacin; or take 100–500 mg per day of niacinamide.

Vitamin B_6: When needed, take an additional 50–200 mg per day.

Calcium: In the form of carbonate or citrate, take 1,000–1,500 mg per day.

Vitamin C: 6,000–18,000 mg per day; take more or less as desired.

Vitamin D: 1,000–2,000 IU per day.

Magnesium: In the form of citrate or gluconate, take 400–600 mg per day or more as needed.

Selenium: 55–200 mcg a day.

Multivitamin: Take a multivitamin twice a day, too. Look for one that also contains 15–30 mg of zinc.

Unless you start taking 100 or more milligrams a day, it is unlikely that you will experience any side effects,[73] but it helps to always take your zinc with food. Being on the pill makes it all the more likely that you need more, not less, of this mineral, so taking 30–50 mg per day would not be too much.

DO WHAT IS BEST FOR YOU

The pill is a drug and no mistake—and in my opinion, a dangerous one. However, I know many women who take the pill and are extremely happy with their choice to do so. I also know many women who have suffered for years with the consequences of that choice. The moral of the story is: do what is best for you. If you happen to be one who is afflicted, like so many women, with adverse side effects, maybe it's time to make a change. Remember: these are not life-saving drugs. You don't *need* them. There are other forms of birth control.

RECOMMENDED READING

Challem, J. *The Food Mood Solution*. Hoboken, NJ: John Wiley & Sons, 2007.

Dean, C. *Hormone Balance: A Woman's Guide to Restoring Health and Vitality*. Avon, MA: Adams Media, 2005.

CHAPTER 7

URINARY TRACT INFECTIONS

"A woman is like a tea bag—only in hot water do you realize how strong she is."
—NANCY REAGAN

Biology, once again, has been unfair: women are far more likely to get urinary tract infections (UTIs) than guys are.[1] Not only are we more likely to get them, we probably will. Half of us will end up with at least one UTI,[2] and about one in four of us will end up with yet another.[3] Since UTIs happen to be one of the most common bacterial infections, millions of gals will end up in the doctor's office each year while the fellas are home, happy and infection-free, and peeing comfortably.[4] Since it is very likely that we will get a UTI, let's take some time to figure out how to get rid of them and, better yet, how to avoid acquiring one in the first place.

JUST WHAT ARE THEY?

It all starts when bad microorganisms work their way into the opening of the urethra and begin multiplying. In 80–85 percent of cases the culprit is *Escherichia coli (E. coli),* a typical inhabitant of our colon.[5] When these trouble-making bacteria set up shop in our urethra, we get a UTI. If the bacteria continue to multiply and move up the ureter (urinary) highway, we now have a bladder infection known as cystitis. If the bacteria continue to travel they can infect our kidneys, resulting in pyelonephritis, a serious kidney infection. It can go from bad to worse, to much worse, so our best bet is to pay close attention to our body, as always. Note any symptoms that may indicate a UTI and address them immediately. It's best to stop the bacteria before they have a chance to further infiltrate our system and cause a more severe infection.

UTI SYMPTOMS

What are the telltale signs of a UTI? Are you reading this chapter in your bathroom, perhaps? If you find yourself constantly having the urge to pee but can't, or very little comes out when you do; if it burns or stings when you urinate or if you have urine that looks milky or cloudy, you may have a urinary tract infection.[6] Other symptoms that may indicate a more serious problem such as a bladder or kidney infection include reddish urine (indicating blood), shakiness, fever, vomiting, chills, nausea, lower abdominal pain or pressure, back or side pain, weight loss, and malaise (that general feeling of "blah"). Treated right away, a UTI is unlikely to do too much damage. Left unchecked, it can become a more serious problem for your urinary tract and kidneys.[7] If you are pregnant, a UTI not only increases your risk for a kidney infection, but also premature delivery of your baby, and sometimes even death to the unborn infant.[8] This is very scary stuff which, of course, we want to avoid. If you think you have a UTI or a more serious infection, get thee to thy doctor! He or she will listen to your symptoms and will most likely do a simple urine test to see if you have a UTI, bladder, or kidney infection. You can even buy a UTI test without a prescription, but you should be in contact with your doctor nonetheless. Continue reading, too.

Risk Factors

Ever heard of "honeymoonitis"? If you are doing what most folks do on their honeymoon (whether you are still honeymooning or not), you have an increased risk for a urinary tract infection. So why do *we* get UTIs when we have sex and men usually don't? Women happen to be prime candidates for UTIs for couple of reasons. *E. coli* is more likely to infiltrate our system because sources of bacteria, our anus and vagina, are geographically closer to our urethra. We also happen to have a shorter urethra, which allows bacteria to get into our bladder sooner.[9] Other contributing factors include having diabetes (which weakens the immune system and makes it harder for your body to fight off illness), not drinking enough fluids, poor hygiene such as not wiping front to back, deodorant sprays and powders, douching, diaphragm use, spermicide use, failing to urinate after sex, loss of estrogen, use of a catheter, and pregnancy.[10] Many of these risk factors can be eliminated to help reduce the chance that you will end up with a UTI.

ANTIBIOTIC TREATMENT

If you get a urinary tract infection (or one of their more serious relatives, such as bladder and kidney infections), your doctor will prescribe antibiotics to cure it. Antibiotics are supposed to kill the bacteria that caused the infections, but these malicious microbes are becoming more resistant to antibiotic therapy. In the United States and overseas, studies are showing increased bacterial resistance to commonly prescribed antibiotics like ampicillin, also known as Principen, Omnipen, Omnipen-N, Totacillin-N, and trimethoprim/sulfamethoxazole (TMP/SMX), marketed as Bactrim, Septra, Cotrim, or Uroplus.[11] We're not talking about something insignificant here. According to these studies, large percentages of the bacteria that cause UTIs are not sensitive to these antibiotics. Additionally, bacteria found to be resistant to one drug are often resistant to many,[12] further complicating treatment. Usually stronger antibiotics are prescribed, but the result is not always favorable.

If you had a UTI (or worse), took antibiotics, and either failed to get better or experienced a recurrence, you know all too well what I'm talking about. About one in four women will have a recurrence within six months of treatment;[13] and most women will experience a second UTI within a year.[14] Notably, women who have recently used antibiotics are at a greater risk for an infection that is now resistant to TMP/SMX.[15] Increased use of antibiotics means more resistant bacteria, and more resistant bacteria means infections that are harder to cure with any antibiotic, the primary medicine your doctor's black bag. Plus, the good bacteria are getting annihilated by antibiotic treatment. Antibiotics, effective (at least initially) at killing off those bad microorganisms, are not selective. An exploding bomb does not know the difference between a munitions factory and a public library. These drugs also kill the good guys, the same good bacteria that help keep your urogenital system healthy. This might further explain why UTI recurrence rates are high after drug treatment.

So, what is the cause of the new, recurrent UTI? Is it the failure of an antibiotic to kill all the bad microbes? Well, if it is, should we take something stronger, more expensive, and more dangerous? Or, as a preventive measure, should we just keep taking antibiotics in order to deliver a constant stream of poison to suppress microbial trouble makers?

Wait a minute. Those choices don't sound that great.

IF YOU CHOOSE TO TAKE ANTIBIOTICS

Depending on the seriousness of your infection, you and your doctor may decide that an antibiotic army is what is needed to start bombing out bad bacteria. *Don't let the antibiotics go it alone.* You should continually introduce good microorganisms back into your ecosystem by ingesting yogurt. Suggested dose: half a cup of plain, unsweetened yogurt every day, now and after your infection is gone. Probiotics like those found in yogurt may help antibiotics do their job better by reducing the risk of opportunistic infections, by creating an environment less hospitable to bad bacteria and by enhancing vaginal immunity to infection.[18] You should also make a point to enhance your immune system by eating right, juicing vegetables, drinking enough water, and taking your vitamins, especially vitamin C. Learn more in the "What To Start Doing" sections of this chapter.

Antibiotics aren't exactly the easy way out. In addition to the widely recognized issue of bacterial tolerance to these drugs, antibiotics used to treat UTIs come fully equipped with side effects. Traditionally prescribed UTI antibiotics like TMP/SMX, nitrofurantoin, and ampicillin may cause upset stomach, vomiting, nausea, headache, severe allergic reactions, and they increase your chances of getting a yeast infection, to name only a few of the nasty outcomes that can result from antibiotic use.[16] If TMP/SMX doesn't work for you, your doctor might prescribe something stronger like a broad-spectrum fluoroquinolone antibiotic such as Ciprofloxacin (Cipro). Cipro, often indicated for bladder and kidney infection, can cause a similar disturbing list of potential adverse effects, as well as tendon rupture.[17] Ouch! Side effects can be dangerous, and are certainly no fun; and it is even less fun to take an antibiotic and experience discomfort, only to find out it didn't work and you still have an uncured UTI.

WHAT TO START DOING

There are many natural, effective, drug-free alternatives to help you prevent urinary tract infections and treat the one you're currently fighting.

For starters, avoid using deodorant sprays and powders, and spermicides, all of which can upset the balance of friendly bacteria in your vagina and the surrounding area. The same goes for douching. Diaphragms are another no-no if you struggle with UTIs. Women who use a diaphragm are two to three times more likely to experience recurrent UTIs than nonusers as it can irritate the surface of your vagina and allow unwanted microbes to adhere to it.[19]

Get a cushy toilet seat. You should visit your restroom more often for the right reason: because you are drinking lots of water. Exactly how much is "a lot" happens to be up to you, although the popular guideline of drinking six to eight eight-ounce glasses seems to be a good recommendation. You may want to drink more if you are in the process of getting over an infection or when you are talking excessively, living in a hot climate, sweating, working out, and so on, but your thirst will probably tell you that anyway! Mind you, coffee and soda do not count as water just because they contain water. Water is water. Much of what we can add to water to make it tastier or more appealing is laden with sugar (real or artificial), caffeine, or other additives. I guess water isn't all that exciting for some folks. It has been reported that one in ten of us drink *no water at all* and half of us just don't drink enough.[20] Water should be the first thing we reach for when we want a drink. Our bodies are made mostly of water; doesn't it just make sense?

When you have to go, *go*! Holding onto urine in the bladder for long periods of time increases your risk for infection.[21]

Urinate after sex. You want any bacteria that can be (or already may be) pushed up in there to be washed out. This prevention technique alone may help rid you of ever having a UTI again.

Wipe front to back. There's no need to put *E. coli* right where it doesn't belong.

Go "number two" often. There's no need to store all that crap up in there. Keep the toxins flowing out freely to avoid putting undue stress on your bladder and kidneys.

Wear cotton underwear. Warm, moist environments are places where bacteria thrive. Don't give 'em an opportunity.

Eat yogurt, at least half a cup a day. Get the good bacteria back in your system where they need to be. *This is especially important during and after antibiotic treatment.*

Juice. Buying a juicer and actually using it are two things that will greatly improve your health in many ways, but for starters, it's an awesome way to combat stubborn UTIs and keep them from coming back. I can't recommend this enough, and yet this might be the routine hardest for you to start doing. It can be time-consuming to make juice, and you have to buy a juicer and all those fresh veggies all the time! But you will notice that once you start juicing regularly you will feel better, and you will notice yourself getting healthier too.

Get your cranberries. Very safe, natural, and well-tolerated by patients, cranberry juice and cranberry tablets have been shown to help prevent recurrent UTIs in women.[22] The science behind it suggests that ingesting cranberry juice or tablets may help keep *E. coli* from sticking to the inside layer of your urinary tract.[23] In a sense,

CRANBERRY JUICE—OR IS IT?

Before you buy, read the label carefully. It is likely that when you purchase cranberry juice at the grocery store, you are paying mostly for water and sugar. "Cranberry juice cocktail" is loaded with sweeteners (real or artificial) and contains less than 30 percent cranberry juice. Be aware, too, of products called "cranberry beverage" and even ones that claim to be 100 percent juice, as only part of that concoction is cranberry-based. These juices may taste nice, but you are getting a whole bunch of sugar you don't really need, and not much of the cranberry that you do. Pure, unadulterated, 100 percent cranberry juice really doesn't taste that great, and therefore, it isn't a popular choice at the supermarket. In fact, you may need to go to a natural foods store to find it. To make the beverage more tolerable, you can dilute it yourself with water. This way, you also avoid the sugar so many of the popular brands contain.

you make the lining more "slippery," and nasty little *E. coli* have nothing to grip, adhere to, multiply on, and use as a home base to grow an infection. It is suggested that you drink three eight-ounce glasses a day of unsweetened cranberry juice as you heal.[24] Read the label. Almost all "cranberry juices" in the supermarket are sweetened. Check online or at the health food store to get the real deal: unsweetened. Continue periodic consumption to help prevent future infections. There are also cranberry pills on the market, for those of you who want to skip the juice but seek the protective benefit of cranberries in a convenient form.

THE VITAMIN SOLUTION

Take vitamin C. Folks, if you have an infection, *the very first thing you should do is load up on vitamin C.* I'm not talking a couple of extra oranges either. I'm talking about taking *grams* (thousands of milligrams) of C, up to "bowel tolerance." Bowel tolerance is exactly what you think it is: the amount your body can handle until you get

WHAT ABOUT ESTROGEN CREAMS?

Estrogen helps keep the lining of the urethra slick, so mean little microbials have a harder time taking hold. Hormonal changes, namely the lowering of estrogen in our system as experienced during our natural cycle or during menopause, may trigger UTIs. A couple of studies found that using vaginal estrogen cream helped reduce the recurrence of urinary tract infections.[25] Even though some women may tolerate this treatment well, there are many possible side effects that make this treatment option not so alluring: vaginal irritation, dizziness, upset stomach, headache, bloating, nausea, weight changes, breast tenderness, changes in sexual appetite, mood swings, possible loss or blurring of vision, trouble breathing, chest pain, various allergic reactions like rash, swelling, and itching, and so on.[26] It may be worth trying a safe, natural alternative first, before turning to estrogen cream.

to saturation or loose bowels. Vitamin C is enormously effective when it comes to treating infection, but you can't be shy. If you are fighting a urinary, bladder, or kidney infection, take a day or two off of work and start downing 2,000–5,000 milligrams (mg) of vitamin C every half an hour. Once you have loose bowels, cut back. Now take 2,000–5,000 mg every hour to two hours. Your therapeutic, bowel tolerance level of vitamin C will depend on your body weight and just how sick you are. Maintain your high level of C, taking just enough to feel better but not enough to cause diarrhea. Over that day and the next you may find you can decrease your dosage still further, until it doesn't take much more than one to two doses of 5,000 mg to get you on the toilet. Yes, your tummy may rumble. Yes, you will feel bloated and gassy temporarily. But your body is now *effectively* fighting the infection without drugs and without dangerous side effects. I know, being at the saturation level of C sometimes isn't the most enjoyable experience, but you'll find that you do *feel better,* even while you are bloated and gassy, and you will *be better* on the inside.

Remember, a lot of C isn't *a lot of* C until you reach bowel tolerance.

Sometimes my friends shy away from therapeutic doses of C because they don't like having to be near a bathroom all day. They don't like that "full" feeling, and passing gas all the time is embarrassing. But ladies, these side effects are harmless and temporary. You are curing a beast of an infection, you are building your immunity at the same time, and you are doing it naturally and relatively quickly. Heck, you have to take some antibiotics for seven to ten days, if you are lucky and they work the first time. If you choose to take antibiotics like your doctor will recommend, you may find that the antibiotic alone is not enough to get rid of a stubborn infection. That's where vitamin C comes in. See C do better! If you are interested in learning more about vitamin C, its history and its use, check out *How to Live Longer and Feel Better* by Linus Pauling, and *Vitamin C: The Real Story* by Steve Hickey and Andrew W. Saul (noted in the recommended reading section at the end of this chapter).

Vitamin A enhances immunity and should be a big part of your battle against UTIs. Your need for vitamin A is higher when you have

JENNIE'S STORY

Jennie's UTI had become a horribly painful kidney infection, and even after being given strong antibiotics, she was still experiencing symptoms of a urinary infection, which is exactly what started the whole mess. Jennie was wondering how she was ever going to get better. The drugs just weren't getting the job done. The next step was hospitalization. How could this be? It was a scary feeling to find out that even doctors really didn't have the "answer." Jennie decided she needed an alternative, and she chose a natural one. She started juicing, carrots mostly, and drinking a liquid pint of them every day. Within the week, her symptoms faded. Now, this was interesting. Once cured, she decided to continue to juice several times a week because, darn it, she just felt *better*. That was seven years ago. Jennie hasn't had a UTI, bladder, or kidney infection since. Not one.

THE RIGHT PILLS TO TREAT A UTI

Give your body the tools it needs to fight your UTI and keep it from coming back. Here's a list of vitamins you'll want to start taking today, and every day. Remember to divide your doses and take these supplements with food.

TO HELP GET RID OF A UTI

Vitamin C: 2,000–5,000 mg *every fifteen minutes to half an hour* until you reach saturation and have loose bowels; then cut back. Take enough C to maintain just-below-saturation levels until all UTI symptoms are gone; this may take more than one day. Then, decrease intake to your daily maintenance dose.

Vitamin A: 10,000–25,000 IU per day in the form of beta-carotene *and drink fresh carrot juice,* one to two pints per day, until symptoms are gone.

Vitamin E: 400–800 IU per day in the form of d-alpha tocopherol.

B Vitamins: 25–50 mg twice a day of B_1, B_2, B_3, and B_6, 25–50 mcg of B_{12}, and 400 mcg of folic acid.

Multivitamin: take two or three times a day in addition to the vitamins listed above.

TO HELP PREVENT UTIS

Vitamin C: 6,000–18,000 mg per day or more or less as needed.

Vitamin A: 5,000–25,000 IU per day in the form of beta-carotene; keep juicing carrots, one to three pints per week.

Vitamin E: 400–800 IU per day in the form of mixed tocopherols or d-alpha tocopherol.

B Vitamins: 25–50 mg once or twice a day of B_1, B_2, B_3, and B_6, 25–50 mcg of B_{12}, and 400 mcg of folic acid.

Multivitamin: take twice daily in addition to your other vitamins.

a serious infection, and even a mild deficiency of A can increase your chance of getting an infection in the first place.[27] The safest, healthiest way to get vitamin A into your system is through beta-carotene, a super-safe form of vitamin A. This can be done with vegetable juicing, especially carrots. Even in huge amounts, beta-carotene is nontoxic.[28] When you can't juice, a daily maintenance dose of 5,000 to 25,000 international units (IU) of vitamin A, via beta-carotene capsules, is a good alternative. While you fight your infection, juice *and* take 5,000–10,000 IU of beta-carotene vitamin A each day.

You should limit your intake of the *fish oil* form of vitamin A, especially if you are pregnant or want to become pregnant as high amounts of vitamin A are associated with birth defects (but so is vitamin A deficiency).[29] The safest bet is to stick with eating and juicing foods high in beta-carotene. Your body will convert beta-carotene into vitamin A in just the right amount your body requires, avoiding any chance of an overdose. You simply cannot hurt yourself, or hurt a developing baby, by eating lots of sweet potatoes, yams, carrots, pumpkin, winter squash, cantaloupe and green leafy vegetables!

Vitamin E deficiency is associated with an increased risk of infection, and supplementation will enhance your immune response and resistance.[30] Start taking 400 to 800 IU a day now and continue after your infection is treated. Look for the all-natural form of E: d-alpha tocopherol. You'll find it is more expensive than other forms of E, but your body will find it more effective and therefore more worth the money.

The B vitamins are also important. Deficiencies of riboflavin (B_2), pantothenic acid (B_5), pyridoxine (B_6), and folic acid (B_9), all negatively affect your body's immune system.[31] B_{12} deficiency increases the likeliness of infection, while supplementation has been found to improve immunity,[32] and niacin (B_3) will help battle your emotional symptoms and stress.[33] Since bladder cancer has been linked to chronic bladder inflammation caused by urinary tract infections,[34] it is good to know that B_6 also helps reduce bladder cancer risk.[35] In fact, patients with bladder cancer who took high doses of vitamins A, C, E, B_6, and the mineral zinc had a 40 percent reduction in bladder cancer tumor recurrence.[36] This also suggests that vitamins work

NOBODY IS DYING
FROM TAKING VITAMINS

In 2008, according to The American Association of Poison Control Centers, there was not even one death from vitamins, minerals, amino acids, or herbs. *Not one.*[37] The same was true for 2009.[38] A 2011 article from the Orthomolecular Medicine News Service highlights this fact:

There was not even one death caused by a dietary supplement in 2009, according to the most recent information collected by the U.S. National Poison Data System.

The new 200-page annual report of the American Association of Poison Control Centers, published in the journal *Clinical Toxicology,* shows zero deaths from multiple vitamins; zero deaths from any of the B vitamins; zero deaths from vitamins A, C, D, or E; and zero deaths from any other vitamin.

Additionally, there were no deaths whatsoever from any amino acid, herb, or dietary mineral supplement.

Two people died from non-nutritional mineral poisoning, one from a sodium salt and one from an iron salt or iron. On page 1139, the AAPCC report specifically indicates that the iron fatality was not from a nutritional supplement. One other person is alleged to have died from an "Unknown Dietary Supplement or Homeopathic Agent." This claim remains speculative, as no verification information was provided.

60 poison centers provide coast-to-coast data for the U.S. National Poison Data System, "one of the few real-time national surveillance systems in existence, providing a model public health surveillance system for all types of exposures, public health event identification, resilience response and situational awareness tracking."

Over half of the U.S. population takes daily nutritional

supplements. Even if each of those people took only one single tablet daily, that makes 155,000,000 individual doses per day, for a total of nearly 57 billion doses annually. Since many persons take more than just one vitamin or mineral tablet, actual consumption is considerably higher, and the safety of nutritional supplements is all the more remarkable.

If nutritional supplements are allegedly so "dangerous," as the FDA and news media so often claim, then *where are the bodies?*[39]

You can subscribe, free of charge, to the Orthomolecular Medicine News Service at http://orthomolecular.org/subscribe.html and access the article archive at http://orthomolecular.org/resources/omns/index.shtml.

best as a team. If you are wondering which B-complex to take, I have found that potency may differ between brands. You should compare bottles and make sure you are getting your money's worth. Take a B-complex twice a day that has 25–50 mg of B_1, B_2, B_3, B_6, B_{12} and 400 micrograms (mcg) of folic acid (once at breakfast and again at lunchtime, in addition to your multivitamin). The B vitamins are water-soluble and very safe, so you can try a B-complex to see if it is right for you, and you needn't worry about doing yourself any harm.

Don't forget to take a multivitamin, too. This is a great way to get a wide variety of the nutrients you require in addition to the megadoses you'll be taking specifically to treat your UTI.

YOUR CHOICE

Many studies show just how ineffective antibiotics can be, but they're the only thing you will be handed if you go to your doctor for help with your UTI discomfort. Many ladies suffer from recurrent infections, but the only treatment in a doctor's medicine bag for UTI, preventive or otherwise, is an antibiotic.

You will find that some critics are quick to point out that natural alternatives shouldn't be recommended. They agree that, yes, vitamins and other natural remedies can be beneficial, but any promising indications will need to be confirmed by more research before doctors can suggest them to their patients. In a sense, they attempt to point out that natural cures aren't always reliable. (Well, *apparently*, neither are antibiotics!) The pharmaceutical-medical profession prefers "standardization of dosages" when we know perfectly well that when it comes to natural cures, dosages have to be adjusted based on how individuals respond, how they *feel*. You can and must approach natural treatment differently. There isn't one dose, one pill, one amount that will do the trick for every person, every time. We have to dislodge ourselves from the medical mindset we are so used to: that we can't and shouldn't attempt to treat our illness on our own because it could be dangerous. With drugs of course, that happens to be true, because they can be dangerous. With *safe,* natural alternatives, we can and often should doctor ourselves.

Admittedly, natural cures require us to be informed to be sure their usage *is* safe. We need to take control of our health and work from many angles to combat illness. Natural cures ask that you start or change many of your lifestyle behaviors if you expect to get better. Natural cures require that you carry out several immunity-building, infection prevention protocols. You need to drink lots of water, *and* juice vegetables regularly, *and* take C, *and* eat yogurt, *and* drink cranberry juice, *and* pay close attention to hygiene. I guess what I am suggesting isn't easy. But isn't suffering from sickness harder? You must trust yourself and trust in your body. You can get better. You will get better. You must work at it. There is no magic pill; the epic failure of antibiotic cures for UTI is evidence of that. You must decide that you will take control of your own body, as so many women have, and treat yourself naturally, safely, and successfully.

It's a pretty good feeling to know that you are capable of treating your own sickness without as much, or even any, pharmaceutical medication. It's a pretty good feeling to *not need to* go to the doctor. Sure, not every disease can be combated at home, but a whole heck of a lot of them can.

Natural cures have several advantages, namely safety and lower cost. If something is safe to try, is inexpensive, and has helped people prevent and treat illness, then shouldn't it be recommended? The key word here is *safe*. It would be a real shame to keep safe, natural health recommendations out of the minds of the public, and yet this is exactly what some studies suggest.

I challenge you to think differently.

RECOMMENDED READING

Hickey, S., A. W. Saul. *Vitamin C: The Real Story, the Remarkable and Controversial Healing Factor.* Laguna Beach, CA: Basic Health Publications, 2008.

Pauling, L. *How to Live Longer and Feel Better.* Corvallis, OR: Oregon State University Press, 2006.

CHAPTER 8

ENDOMETRIOSIS

"We must not, in trying to think about how we can make a big difference, ignore the small daily differences we can make which, over time, add up to big differences that we often cannot foresee."
—MARIAN WRIGHT EDELMAN

Endometriosis is another scary term in our women's ailment dictionary. We might learn about it from a friend or family member; we may be looking into its causes and treatments because we are worried we are going to get it. For some of us, that fear is already a reality, and our relationships, our job, and our social life suffer because of it. We may be experiencing tremendous pain. We may be tired. We may be suffering inconvenient bleeding. We may even have trouble getting pregnant.

JUST WHAT IS IT?

Each month, when we have that pleasant experience we call our period, the lining of our uterus (the endometrium) sheds. Naturally, this is normal and expected. However, sometimes endometrial cells show up in places in our bodies where they should not be. They can turn up in such inconvenient spots as the outer surface of our uterus, ovaries, or fallopian tubes, or in the lining of our pelvis, intestines, bladder, cervix, or vagina.

These misplaced cells respond to our menstrual cycle in the same way the cells inside our uterus do: they build and then shed. But once they shed, they have no place to go. Instead of moseying out of our bodies with the rest of our period, these discarded cells cause inflammation, scar tissue, cysts (little sacs of fluid), bowel and bladder problems, and from these, pain.

Symptoms

If we have symptoms, it is usually pain, and lots of it. Women with endometriosis may be experiencing painful sex, painful bowel movements, pain when urinating, lower back pain, and painful abdominal and menstrual cramps. We may also experience fatigue or abnormal bleeding such as a heavy menstrual flow or spotting between periods, or we may have trouble getting pregnant. However, some of us with endometriosis will not notice any symptoms at all. Doctors may diagnose endometriosis by doing something as simple as a pelvic exam or perhaps an ultrasound or MRI. To be absolutely sure, they will do a surgical procedure called a laparoscopy to look for scar tissue, cysts, or tissue implants.

How Do You Get It?

Well, nobody really knows, which is not very reassuring I know, but it is estimated to affect some 3 to 18 percent of women in the United States.[1] There seem to be several things that may increase or decrease our risk of endometriosis, even if we aren't particularly sure how we get it in the first place.

POSSIBLE RISK FACTORS

If you happen to be a woman of childbearing age, that's a risk factor for endometriosis. Estrogen appears to make the problem worse, and that may be why patients and doctors so often turn to hormonal birth control to help manage estrogen and, consequently, help manage symptoms. Hormonal birth control suppresses ovulation. In turn, it

ENDOMETRITIS (NOT TO BE CONFUSED WITH ENDOMETRIOSIS)

Endometr*itis*, although it may sound similar, is different from endo-metri*osis*. Endometritis is when the lining of your uterus becomes inflamed or irritated. In other words, it is an endometrial infection. You may have symptoms such as abnormal vaginal bleeding or dis-charge, malaise (feeling "blah" all over), abdominal pain, abdom-inal swelling, and fever.[2] It happens to be the most common cause of fever experienced postpartum.[3] This illness can be caused by several factors. One way of getting it is through sexually transmit-ted diseases (another good reason to only have protected sex), but it can also be caused by imbalances in your normal vaginal bacte-ria or an infection that moves up from your lower genital tract. It can also occur after miscarriage. However, is most likely to happen after childbirth, especially Caesarean section deliveries.

Here are a few hints to help prevent and treat infections naturally:

1. Practice safe sex.

2. Don't douche. Women who have endometritis or upper genital tract infections were more likely to have douched more than once a month as compared to women who did not have these illnesses.[4] Douching may give you the feeling of being clean, but it really is not helping. It disturbs the natural balance of bac-teria in your vagina. For example, women who douche are more likely to get bacterial vaginosis.[5] Bacterial vaginosis (BV) hap-pens to be associated with endometritis.[6] Furthermore, women with endometritis are less likely to have certain *Lactobacillus* species present,[7] which is a condition found in BV patients as well. This is a problem you can help fix. To help prevent and treat BV and reduce your risk of endometritis, instead of flush-ing out the area, reintroduce good bacteria (probiotics) to your system by eating half a cup of plain yogurt every day. If you think you have BV, check out Chapter 4 in this book for more targeted advice.

3. Antibiotics may not have all the answers. Preventing your infection or killing off one you have with antibiotics may create bacterial imbalances and contribute to other problems caused by eliminating the good bacteria along with the bad. Since antibiotics do not kill selectively, if you choose to take them, fight to keep the good guys working for you by regularly introducing probiotics and by taking your vitamins to keep your immune system strong.

4. If we are talking about infections, then we should also be talking about vitamin C. If you have an infection, take enough C to reach bowel tolerance. Keep with it until your symptoms are gone, and gradually reduce your megadose to a maintenance dose, which is the amount you should be taking anyway, to help keep your immune system strong. Other immunity builders, such as vitamins A and E are also worth taking to help battle an infection.

is thought to lessen the building, bleeding, and shedding of your endometrium and help keep endometriosis implants from growing.

Alcohol Consumption

Could alcohol consumption be a contributing risk factor for endometriosis? Some researchers think so. Grodstein and colleagues analyzed the drinking habits of over 4,500 women and concluded "[t]he risk of endometriosis was roughly 50% higher in case subjects with any alcohol intake than in control subjects."[8] They noted "[a] change in estrogen levels with alcohol intake appears to us to be a likely explanation for any increased risk. We also found an elevated risk of ovulatory infertility with alcohol use, and there is increasing evidence that moderate alcohol drinking may be associated with breast cancer; these are all estrogen-related disorders."[9]

Caffeine

Like so many things, I have seen it argued both ways, but it has been shown that a high intake of caffeine is associated with an increased risk of endometriosis and infertility due to endometriosis.[10] Taking in 300 milligrams (mg) a day or more seems to be an issue.[11] Figure there is about 100 mg of caffeine in a six-ounce cup of coffee, but that can vary pretty significantly. Since infertility may be one of the most unpleasant side effects of endometriosis, it makes sense to cut your caffeine intake, especially if you want to get pregnant.

Bad Diet

Eating a nutrient-deficient diet is never a good idea. For example, women who have a diet high in trans fats (those unhealthy fats often found in junk foods) have a greater risk of being diagnosed with endometriosis.[12] Common sense would tell you that a bad diet is certainly not going to help you avoid getting or treating a condition like endometriosis. To prevent, manage, or cure any disease, you have to be willing to give your body the right foods, vitamins, and minerals.

Other Factors

Other risk factors for endometriosis include your family history (does your mom or sister have it?), getting your period at an early age, having menstrual periods that last longer than seven days and/or cycles that are less than twenty-seven days, having menstrual cramps (which could be a cause or a symptom), and never having given birth.[13]

WHAT THE DOCTOR MAY SAY

Ladies, even though there is no "cure" for endometriosis, the doctor's handbag is full of all sorts of medicines that he or she will be happy to dispense and procedures that he or she will be willing to perform. These will do all sorts of things to your body except, perhaps, get rid of the disease for good. Conventional treatments will attempt to suppress symptoms, alter your body's hormones, or remove the implants through the use of pain relievers, hormonal therapies, or surgery, respectively. Your choice of treatment will depend on your own personal symptoms, your age, and your fertility plans. Are your symptoms mild or severe? Are children in your future? What makes the most sense for you now? No matter what your personal situation, conventional treatment is an option, but in many cases it's a pretty drastic measure. Read on and see what you think.

Let's start with the least scary choice. Your doctor may suggest that you take pain relievers for the pain associated with endometriosis, particularly anti-inflammatory pain meds like ibuprofen or naproxen to help reduce inflammation, pain, and bleeding. Unfortunately, these will not work for one in five of us.[14] It is also not advisable to take these if you want to become pregnant, and for those of us with sensitive tummies, it may be uncomfortable to continuously down pain killers. Still, anti-inflammatory pain relief may be a less invasive option than other conventional treatments for endometriosis.

Doctors are likely to suggest using hormonal birth control pills to manage the discomforts of endometriosis or try to stop it from getting worse. Obviously, you cannot use this treatment if you want to get pregnant, and the pain can come back once you stop using hormonal birth control.[15] It is argued that the side effects from the pill are not as severe as other forms of hormone therapy, but there still are plenty to contend with. Check out Chapter 6 in this book for more information.

There are other forms of hormone therapy to control pain and shrink endometrial implants, including progestogens (progestins), gonadotropin-releasing hormone (GnRH) analogues, Danazol (a derivative of the synthetic steroid ethisterone), aromatase inhibitors, and Mirena, an anintrauterine device (IUD). Unfortunately, many women will decide that the side effects of these treatments are intolerable. They can cause osteoporosis, a slew of menopausal symptoms, and endometriosis pain symptoms can come back once treatment is discontinued.[16] Plus, hormone treatment does not always work even while you are on it.

The same laparoscopy that may be used to ultimately determine whether or not you have endometriosis is also a vehicle for removal of implants, cysts, or scar tissue. Getting these unwanted residents out of you may reduce the pain you are experiencing and allow for pregnancy. It is not a cure-all; endometriosis can come back. But for women that want to get pregnant, this is pretty much the only option conventional medicine has to offer.

The U.S. National Library of Medicine (National Institutes of Health) states "[h]ormone therapy and laparoscopy cannot cure endometriosis. However, these treatments can help relieve some or all symptoms in many women for years."[17] I guess that should be encouraging, but I find it hard to get excited about drug therapies and surgery that just postpone symptoms for a few years, especially when the side effects, notably those of hormonal treatments, can be so awful. It makes one wonder: is the treatment worse than the disease?

Lastly, there is the most drastic move of all: hysterectomy. Some women will choose major surgery and have their uterus and ovaries completely removed in order to treat endometriosis. Of course, if you want to become pregnant, this is not an option for you, and even a hysterectomy does not guarantee that endometriosis will not reoccur![18]

With a failure rate of conventional treatments ranking somewhere around 20–25 percent,[19] it is no surprise that some of us are looking for other ways to cure this "incurable" disease. Pills, drugs, invasive surgery . . . I suppose if they worked, they could be worth the side effects and discomfort. I look at it this way: conventional treatment is always available, but wouldn't it be nice to manage our symptoms without having to take hormones or go under the knife? It makes sense to try safe, nutritional alternatives, especially if they help!

WHAT TO START DOING

I do not think it is much of a solution to simply cover up the symptoms of endometriosis with a drug that makes you feel worse, or to just submit to the operating table. Of course, all women must do right by themselves, and if you feel these measures are necessary, I am certainly not here to stop you! However, I am here to provide some nutritional alternatives to conventional medicine that will help you feel better, may make surgery less urgent, and even fight infertility without the list of unbearable drug-induced side effects.

Eat Right to Reduce Risk and Reduce Pain

Eating right is always a good idea, but in this case it may even help you from getting endometriosis in the first place. When it comes to diet and the risk of endometriosis, Parazzini et al found "a significant reduction in risk emerged for higher intake of green vegetables and fresh fruit, whereas an increase in risk was associated with high intake of beef and other red meat."[20]

It has always been a good idea to steer away from salt, sugar, animal fats, red meat, caffeine, alcohol, and junk food. But in addition to avoiding these foods, we need to *add* more raw vegetables and fruits. Even health-conscious people may find it difficult to follow the government recommendation regarding the amount of veggies and fruits that should be present in their meals, now suggested to be half of your plate.[21] And it may be even more difficult to eat that amount of *raw* veggies and fruits. Vegetable juicing comes in handy here. It is a great way to get a large quantity of really good-for-you raw food, without even having to chew it all up! In addition, eat whole grains, raw nuts, seeds, fish, and drink plenty of water.

Okay, so nutrition may reduce your risk for getting endometriosis, but what if you already have it? You should still avoid junk and eat lots of raw fruits and vegetables. We are not talking about a hormonal pill, patch, injection, or surgery to experience relief. Instead, we can help ourselves feel better by being mindful of what we put in our bodies. We are going to eat anyway, why not make better choices about what goes down the gullet? Good nutrition can help a woman "tolerate medical treatments, increase her ability to deal with potential side effects of treatment, increase her energy, and enhance her ability to think clearly"[22] all of which sound like positives indeed. One study that looked at 180 women with endometriosis over a six-month period found that 86 percent of the women experienced improvement with their symptoms, notably abdominal pain and infertility, through nutritional therapy.[23] For some of these women, wheat and dairy caused adverse reactions.[24] You may want to consider trying a wheat-free, gluten-free diet. Nutritionist Dian Mills found that pain subsides in eight out of ten endometriosis patients when wheat is removed from the diet.[25]

Good nutrition will help me feel better? Boy, this all sounds so . . . familiar. That is because doctors have been saying it for, like, ever.

Body Therapy for Pain Relief

Being stressed, tired, anxious, depressed, angry, frustrated, or tense can't possibly help you feel less pain. This is where body (and mind) therapy comes in, starting with getting moving, or just taking a break.

Exercise and relaxation techniques may help you alleviate pain due to endometriosis. Exercise reduces stress, and since stress can affect how severe your menstrual pain is,[26] it can help you feel better and burn some calories in the process. Some women may find that other relaxing, stress-reducing activities like massage therapy, acupuncture, and yoga help, too. You do not need to wait for a scientific study to come out to tell you that massage or meditation will help you; if it works for you, do it!

Heat is another means of drug-free pain relief. Two studies on menstrual pain and cramping showed continuous low-level heat wraps were as effective, if not more effective, than acetaminophen and ibuprofen.[27]

Don't underestimate the power of a conversation. Talk about your experiences and frustrations. The emotional support of a girl-to-girl chat has helped many a gal through tough times, and this situation is no different. I'm not saying that talking to somebody will cure your disease, but it can really help you feel better.

As far as I am concerned, everything on that short list is worth trying. It is a start, anyway. I mean, who couldn't use a little more exercise, relaxation, and girl time?

VITAMINS, MINERALS, AND FATTY ACIDS

It's safe to say that if there is no readily available cure for a disease, it may be because the cause of the ailment is nutritional in nature. No drug or hormone will give the body the nutrients it seeks. For women with endometriosis pain, cramps, heavy bleeding, fatigue, and even

MENSTRUAL CRAMPS AND PAIN: PRIMARY AND SECONDARY DYSMENORRHOEA

Primary dysmenorrhoea (the fancy name for menstrual pain and cramping) is called "primary" because it occurs in an otherwise healthy woman. Secondary dysmenorrhoea gets its name because it is secondary to an original condition, such as endometriosis, fibroids, and cysts. All of these are examples of a possible underlying cause of secondary dysmenorrhoea. The difference between the two basically ends there. Whether your pain is caused by endometriosis or common menstrual complaints may not be as important as understanding that the pain symptoms of both are similar if not the same. In other words, a cramp is a cramp.

Is this my excuse for including studies in this chapter that discuss the relief of cramps and menstrual pain in women with primary dysmenorrhoea, even though your condition is technically considered secondary dysmenorrhoea if you have endometriosis? Yes, it is. I think there is great value in looking at natural treatments that help one or both of these conditions. Doctors approach this in a similar way; in either case, they will first recommend that you try pain killers and/or hormonal birth control to manage your symptoms. If endometriosis is confirmed, they may suggest other hormonal drugs, but whether you are taking the pill or following some other hormone protocol, it is pretty much the same solution: manage your hormone production through treatment of your condition with drug-administered hormones. If similar conventional therapies are recommended for both types of dysmenorrhoea, why not do the same with natural therapies? Even if you are diagnosed with endometriosis, there is always the possibility that your pain is being caused by something else, and for that reason alone it is worth looking into all of the natural therapies for dysmenorrhoea rather than simply eliminating studies because "menstrual pain" has been given a different title.

infertility, all are unwelcome symptoms and the drugs just aren't cutting it. Vitamins, minerals, and fatty acids can help. Nutrients can help alleviate what endometriosis makes you suffer through, and boost your immune system, too.

Magnesium and Calcium

Menstrual cramping (dysmenorrhoea) caused by endometriosis is pretty awful. There is really no pleasant way to put it: it feels like you are being punched it the stomach, except the fist is never removed. The pressure and pain can be excruciating. Fortunately, there are natural alternatives that can offer much relief from this menstrual cramping and pain.

Magnesium may help you get rid of cramps,[28] which makes a lot of sense since magnesium deficiency can cause cramping among other unpleasant symptoms.[29] Magnesium also plays a role in muscle relaxation. (Remember those Epsom salt or magnesium sulfate baths Grandma recommended to sooth aching muscles?) Now's also a good time to load up on those healthy foods like nuts, beans, spinach, and other green leafy vegetables, the kind of foods we should already be trying to incorporate into our diet. Even with some close attention to what we eat, it may be difficult to get the United States Recommended Dietary Allowance (RDA) of 310–400 mg per day, and indeed, most women do not.[30] To obtain therapeutic levels of magnesium, supplements may be necessary. Each of us is different, and therefore, our magnesium requirement may be higher, especially if we have cramps. (If you are experiencing any constipation, magnesium can help that, too.) Consider taking 300 mg per day, twice a day, in addition to food sources of magnesium. Supplement your magnesium intake with additional calcium: 600 mg per day or more. It's easier to find calcium in our diets, but you may wish to supplement your intake to get more. Hundreds of women who took 1,200 mg per day of calcium significantly helped reduce premenstrual syndrome (PMS) pain symptoms,[31] so it's worth taking this safe, essential mineral to help battle your condition.

B Vitamins

The B vitamins may be very beneficial in your battle against pain and cramps, and they can help lower your estrogen levels. One study done with over 500 women showed that 87 percent of these ladies completely eliminated mild to severe dysmenorrhoea by taking 100 mg per day of thiamine (B_1) for ninety days, with no side effects.[32]

Niacin (B_3) or in the form of niacinamide (the kind that won't cause flushing, that feeling of being itchy, tingly, and warm all over) may help, too; the suggested dose is 100 mg twice daily.[33] Your body will be more tolerant of niacin if it is taken with vitamin C, which can help reduce flushing. Even though a niacin flush is completely safe, some folks prefer forms of niacin that do not have this side effect.

Another B vitamin worth your attention for the management of dysmenorrhoea is B_6, to the tune of 200 mg per day.[34]

A good B-complex will help get you these Bs as well as all the others, like pantothenic acid (B_5) and folate (B_9).

Iron

If you happen to be suffering from heavy bleeding during your period, iron is a good mineral to be adding back into your system. Even if you are not bleeding buckets, getting at least the RDA of iron is essential for any woman who gets her period, and it may even help with dysmenorrhoea.[35] However, a significant number of American women are not getting enough iron.[36] It is estimated that one in five of ladies of childbearing age suffer from iron-deficiency anemia, which can cause you to feel fatigued, and experience dizziness, cold hands and feet, headaches, shortness of breath, and chest pains.[37] It's not just American gals that need more iron. The Centers for Disease Control and Prevention states that iron deficiency is the most common nutritional deficiency worldwide.[38] Your doctor can check your iron levels; you may want to see where you stand. Iron-rich foods include oysters, clams, and organ meats. If those don't get your mouth watering, iron supplements are always available. Vitamin C helps your body effectively absorb iron, so take it along with your iron supplement and along with meals to get the most out of iron rich foods.

BUILD YOUR IMMUNE SYSTEM

One theory about the cause of endometriosis is that it is due to a weakened immune response. Instead of the immune system destroying any rogue endometrial cells, it is theorized that this does not happen to the extent it should in women with endometriosis.[39] Retrograde menstruation is thought to be a possible cause of endometriosis; this is when the menstrual flow travels up into the body, allowing those endometrial cells to get to places they should not rather than exiting through the uterus. However, retrograde menstruation happens to occur in most women of reproductive age.[40] So, why do some ladies get endometriosis and others do not? Perhaps the key lies in our immune response. It turns out that women with endometriosis are far more likely to have autoimmune conditions like chronic fatigue, hyperthyroidism, rheumatoid arthritis, fibromyalgia, allergies, and asthma.[41] Women with endometriosis are also more likely to report conditions such as recurrent upper respiratory and vaginal infections, and even cancer.[42] Once again, the immune system is not doing as good a job as it should or could. So what can be done about it? A lot. You can use nutrition to build up your immune system so it can better fend off disease. Eat right, drink plenty of water, drink fresh, raw vegetable juice, and take your vitamins.

Vitamin E

Over fifty years ago, it was found that vitamin E could help improve dysmenorrhoea.[43] In a more recent study, taking 200 international units (IU) of vitamin E twice a day helped relive menstrual pain, and it reduced blood loss.[44] It is common to feel fatigued when you are losing blood, so in this case, vitamin E could also help keep you from feeling so worn out. It is difficult to get even just one 200 IU dose of vitamin E in your diet, unless your daily morning beverage consists of several cups of oil or you spread a generous six pounds of peanut butter on that slice of whole wheat toast. You would probably have to get even more creative for the second dose at dinner time. When it comes to vitamin E, a natural supplement is surely the best way to go.

Vitamin C and More

Want to reduce pain and inflammation? Vitamin E and vitamin C were shown to do just that for women with endometriosis. In one study, 1,200 IU of vitamin E and 1,000 mg of vitamin C taken for two months helped forty women experience significant improvement of their endometriosis pain and a reduction in all their inflammatory markers.[45] Five women got pregnant in the vitamin E and C group, so they were excluded from the remainder of the study.[46] In the forty women in the control group, there was no improvement in pain or inflammation, and no one got pregnant.[47] Another recommendation for antioxidant treatment of endometriosis suggests an even higher dose of vitamin C along with a good dose of vitamin E: 2,000 mg of vitamin C, three times a day, and 400 IU-1,000 IU of vitamin E.[48] More promising research out there suggests that the puzzle of endometriosis may be related to a lack of antioxidants like vitamins C and E and to a deficiency in other nutrients, including vitamin A, selenium, and zinc.[49] Supplements may be just what you need to start feeling better, soon.

Selenium

Selenium recharges vitamin E, a nutrient that may help reduce cramping, menstrual pain, and blood loss in women. Since selenium and vitamin E work well together, take them together. You can get some selenium in your diet by eating Brazil nuts, garlic, vegetables, mushrooms, liver, brown rice, whole grains, eggs, and fish, but I recommend that you supplement what you are already ingesting with an additional 100–200 mcg (that's micrograms) of selenium each day.

Fatty Acids

Data suggest that women who consume more omega-3 fatty acids are less likely to be diagnosed with endometriosis.[50] There may also be a link between low levels of omega-3 and infertility.[51] The omega-3 fatty acids taken alone[52] or with B_{12}[53] may help alleviate pain and cramping. This can be because an imbalance between omega-6 fatty acids (readily obtained in our diet) and omega-3 fatty acids (harder to obtain in our diet) is associated with menstrual cramps and pain. The solution? To decrease the likelihood that you'll get endometriosis and to help halt and prevent cramps and pain, focus on getting more of the omega-3 fatty acids in your diet or grab a supplement to make sure you are getting enough even when you can't (or don't want to) load up on items like flaxseeds, walnuts, tuna, salmon, or sardines.

FIGHTING THE WORST OF ENDOMETRIOSIS: NOT BEING ABLE TO CONCEIVE

For those of us who want to have children, infertility is perhaps the most awful possible consequence of endometriosis. Up to 50 percent of women with endometriosis are infertile,[54] which makes this no small matter, especially since so many women have endometriosis. Of course, you are going to want to do everything possible to try and have that baby you have always wanted. "You can't get pregnant" is just not a statement I, you, or any woman needs to accept just yet.

A Medical Perspective

After months and months of disappointment, we will probably turn to our doctors for guidance. Sadly, there isn't a whole lot they can offer for endometriosis-associated infertility. Laparoscopic surgery to remove endometrial implants is just about the only medical treatment available to help increase one's chances of getting pregnant. Other treatments, like hormone therapy, make it unlikely that you will become pregnant while you are being treated and don't seem to help you get pregnant after stopping treatment either.[55] However, even laparoscopy, the conventional treatment option with the most pregnancy potential, might not have all the answers. It may be just as effective in treating endometriosis-associated infertility as doing nothing at all.[56]

Well ladies, if you want children, doing nothing is just not an option.

A Nutritional Perspective

Think about this: is surgical removal of an implant really going to resolve why endometriosis occurs in the first place? Okay, perhaps surgery can remove a physical blockage preventing conception, I'll give you that. But maybe there is a different way to look at treatment for those women who don't have a clear answer as to why they can't

---

YOUR NUTRIENT GUIDE FOR ENDOMETRIOSIS AND ENDOMETRIOSIS-ASSOCIATED INFERTILITY

Here are the nutrients that can help prevent and alleviate symptoms from endometriosis and boost immunity:

B-complex: Take one once or twice a day that contains 25–50 mg each of B_1, B_2, B_3, and B_6, and 400 mcg of folic acid (B_9); the amounts of B_{12}, biotin, and pantothenic acid can vary. Consider taking additional B_1 (to reach 100 mg daily intake), B_3, (to reach 200 mg per day), and B_6 (to get 200 mg per day) in addition to the amounts present in your B-complex.

Vitamin A: Take 5,000–25,000 IU per day of this powerful antioxidant in the form of beta-carotene; or drink all you want of fresh, raw carrot juice; or eat other foods rich in beta-carotene like sweet potatoes, pumpkin, and green leafy veggies.

Calcium: Take 600–1,200 mg per day in the form of carbonate or citrate; take separately from your iron supplement.

conceive. Is it safe to assume that perhaps the body's immune response needs some bolstering, that perhaps more antioxidants are required, that maybe a better diet will help the body heal and repair itself? I would like you to consider that endometriosis-associated infertility may have to do with your body's need for better nutrition. It makes sense that the healthier your body is, the more likely it is that you will be able to have a baby. There are nutritional options you can try right now to safely and actively fight infertility. You can still go ahead and schedule that surgery later, but why not try nutrition first? You have nothing to lose except the inability to have a child.

Diet

If you want to conceive, be as healthy as you can be. This begins with a healthy diet and lifestyle. Nutritional therapy may be just what

Vitamin C: 6,000–18,000 mg per day; take more or less as needed.

Vitamin E: 400–1,200 IU per day in the form of mixed tocopherols (best) or d-alpha tocopherol; take separately from your iron supplement.

Iron: In the form of ferrous fumarate, ferrous gluconate, or carbonyl iron, take 18–27 mg per day; take separately from your vitamin E and calcium supplements.

Magnesium: In the form of citrate or gluconate, take 600 mg per day or more as needed.

Omega-3 fatty acids: Look for a fish oil supplement that contains 900–1,000 mg total of EPA and DHA omega-3 fatty acids. Be sure to read the label. A tablet that contains 1,000 mg of fish oil may only contain 300 mg of omega-3 fatty acids. You will want to take three of those a day to get the optimum dose.

Selenium: 100–200 mcg a day.

Multivitamin: You should also be taking a multivitamin twice a day in addition to all these other vitamins and minerals. Look for one that also contains 15–30 mg of zinc.

you need to increase your chances of conception, even with endometriosis. What does a healthy diet look like? This will probably sound pretty familiar: avoid fried foods, sugar, junk food, excess salt, animal fat, and red meat, and eat plenty of fresh, raw fruits and vegetables. Additionally, some research suggests that alcohol[57] and caffeine[58] (whether you have endometriosis or not[59]) are worth avoiding if you want to become pregnant. It's best to avoid these substances anyway when you are pregnant, so there's no harm, and probably some benefit, in starting early in preparation for that baby. By the way, if you are a smoker (or think you might like to start) add that to the list of no-no's.

Vitamins and Minerals

The promising research that suggests that lower levels of antioxidants may be part of the endometriosis mystery may also help us better understand infertility due to endometriosis.[60] It is encouraging to see that studies done on infertility are getting results with nutritional supplementation. In one small study, women who had attempted to have a baby for six to thirty-six months without success were given a supplement containing vitamin E, zinc, selenium, and iron; they showed a significant increase in ovulation and pregnancy rates.[61] Another study showed that supplementation with 750 mg per day of vitamin C could also increase pregnancy rates.[62] The authors added that vitamin C treatment was "cost-beneficial and does not have side effects."[63] Another study found that women who take multivitamins were less likely to have ovulatory infertility,[64] as were women who took iron supplements.[65] Admittedly, these studies were not specific to women with endometriosis. But here's the thing: if endometriosis could be associated with a lack of proper nutrition and antioxidants, if multiple types of infertility could benefit from proper nutrition and antioxidants,[66] and if women often experience infertility because of endometriosis, it seems to me there is an obvious connection here. Certainly, it does no harm to ensure your body is getting the essential nutrients it needs to try and correct the devastating impact of not being able to have a child when you want one.

For more on infertility, check out the chapter in this book dedicated to the topic.

AN END TO ENDOMETRIOSIS

There is nothing quite as awful as being told you have a disease, except when that news is coupled with being told that there isn't a cure. Even when the disease interferes with life plans, such as having a family, we still try to keep our chin up and hope for a solution.

I say we can do more than hope. We have a choice: to manage symptoms by suppressing them with drugs or surgery, or to make our bodies as healthy as possible so they become inhospitable hosts for sickness. A safe, natural, nutritional approach that helps endometriosis may sound too good to be true, but it is already a reality for those women who have already benefited from such lifestyle changes. Be proactive. Be strong. Keep fighting. Let nutrition help.

CHAPTER 9

INFERTILITY: TROUBLE GETTING AND STAYING PREGNANT

*"I have learned to use the word impossible
with the greatest caution."*
—WERNHER VON BRAUN

Just the word *infertility* can send shivers down one's spine. It sounds so . . . final. But it doesn't always have to be. Okay, so you haven't gotten pregnant, *yet*. Until we look into all that can help out, perhaps infertility should just be called "trouble getting pregnant."

JUST WHAT IS IT?

If you keep on trying and those double lines don't show up on the pregnancy test display, your doctor may use the dreaded term "infertility." He or she may not have sworn at you, but hearing the "I" word is likely to offend even the thickest-skinned of patients. It is a tough word to hear, let alone believe. Even if he or she doesn't say it, the thought lingers in the air. You have been trying for months and months, perhaps well over a year, and nothing has happened. It can turn your whole world on end. To make things worse, it seems every girlfriend of yours is sporting a bump, every shopper in the mall is heading toward the maternity store, and commercial after commercial on TV shows happy couples and ladies with large, blooming bellies. Family pressure can make it even worse. (How do you explain?)

Then there's that dreaded question from anyone and everyone: "So . . . when are you going to have kids?"

Frankly, it is nobody's damn business. But each time you are asked, it just adds to the feverish longing you already have to make a baby. Each time you get your period, it is a slap in the face. Your heart sinks, the tears start, and no matter how your partner may console you, it feels as if you have failed.

"SO WHEN ARE YOU GOING TO HAVE KIDS?"

Before we even delve into the topic, you need to find ways to help protect yourself from (at best) the innocently curious and from (at worst) the downright nosy folks out there. You are putting enough pressure on yourself—you don't need it from anyone else.

I've learned that people can't help themselves. If you haven't had kids, they want to know when you will, and if you have them, they want to know when you will have more. If you have too many, they will comment on that. If you have none at all, they comment on that, too. If you have a boy, they'll ask about when you will try for a girl. It never, never ends. When you are faced with the possibility that you might not be able to get pregnant, it takes such "innocent" questioning to a whole new level. You are not about to tell your coworkers how long you have been trying or about that miscarriage. So, it is time to tell them something else that will shut them up, in a nice way.

My solution is to answer inquisitive individuals in such a way that makes them more uncomfortable than they made me when they asked such a personal question in the first place. Below are some of the responses I have given (or just happen to like) to address the "When are you going to have kids?" question. The truth and tact, of course, are optional. Bravery, however, is not.

- "Wow! That is such a *personal* question. I mean, you are asking me when I am going to have unprotected *sex*. That's really what you want to know, right? When I am going to have *sex* au naturale? That's just so *personal,* you know?" (I gave this answer, rather loudly, I might add, at a family Christmas party, with a grin on my face from ear to ear. I was never asked about babies again, at least not from that bunch.)

- "Ooo! We are still experimenting with the best sexual positions. Last night we tried . . . ." (Insert position of choice with excessive detail.)

- "Until I get over this icky infection (feel free to add details), sex is out of the question! But I'll let you know as soon as we are doing it again!" (Perfect choice for the nosy lunch bunch at work.)

- "I just *love* (insert sexual act that does not involve intercourse), so it makes it harder to get around to making all those babies!"

- "Oh, no worries! We are having sex *all* the time. We just ordered . . . ." (Insert a gasp-worthy video, book, or magazine title. Or describe a sex toy that would make Sue Johanson blush.)

Okay, Okay. I know this is no laughing matter. We will keep it pretty serious from now on, I promise. And, if you prefer, be gracious and polite when faced with the kid question. Just because I reached my wit's end and started doling out quippy comebacks does not mean you need to follow suit.

Why Might I Have It?

Possible reasons behind female infertility are many, including endometriosis, ovulation issues like irregular ovulation, fibroids or cysts that need to be removed, abnormal or blocked fallopian tubes likely caused by pelvic inflammatory disease or endometriosis, hormonal imbalances like hypothyroidism, trouble with immune function, sexually transmitted diseases (STDs), and premature ovarian failure.

When doctors just don't know, unexplained infertility is the term used to describe cases that are otherwise undiagnosed. It is also just as likely that your man could be the one contributing to the infertility issue.

The good news is that there are also dietary, nutritional, and lifestyle factors that play a role in the many possible causes of infertility. This is good news because you and your partner can improve these things right now, together, without the help of your local fertility clinic.

NATURAL APPROACHES TO INFERTILITY

If you are worried that there might be a problem with your (or his) baby-making parts, you and your man should head to the doctor for a checkup. It is very possible that your doctor can help put some pieces of your infertility puzzle together. Of course, there are all sorts of medical treatments, drugs, and surgical procedures available to help a couple try and have the children they always wanted. However, I doubt you are reading this book or this chapter because you want to hear about all the latest technological advances in fertility treatments. It's far more likely that you are interested in how vitamins, diet, and lifestyle can make a difference, so read on.

WHAT TO STOP DOING

Some of the things you can do to help increase the chances you and your partner will be able to conceive are as simple as stopping behaviors that are known to make it harder to become pregnant.

Stop Smoking. Him, Too

With a potential 60 percent overall increase in the risk of infertility in smokers, it makes a whole lot of sense to put the smokes down if you want to get pregnant.[1] Of course, infertility isn't the only health risk of smoking, and it won't do your baby any good once you get pregnant either. So, if you need one more reason to quit, that desire for a baby needs to outweigh your desire to smoke. This doesn't just apply to you; it also applies to your man. Oh, and the "stop smoking" advice also applies to the inhalation of other leafy substances, in other words, marijuana.[2] Once again, that goes for him too.[3]

Stop Drinking. Him, Too

I wonder if there would be as many kids around as there are if folks *weren't* tipping back a few, but believe it or not, alcohol doesn't seem to help you get pregnant. Basically, research suggests that if you want to get pregnant, you may want to skip the drinks.[4] One large study found that even moderate consumption of alcohol (defined by these researchers as one drink or less per day) increased the risk of female infertility by 30 percent.[5] And ladies, the trend for decreased fertility continues the more you drink.[6] For women who are putting down more than seven drinks a week, a 60 percent increase in infertility has been shown.[7] And if your man is a heavy drinker, cutting back will help him be part of the solution, too.

Cut Your Caffeine Intake

Reducing your intake of caffeine, or just staying away from it altogether, may be helpful. A number of studies have suggested that there may be a link between caffeine intake and female infertility.[8] An occasional cup of coffee isn't much of a concern here, but if you *have* to have your morning, noon, and night café latte, it may be time to reevaluate your beverage choices. Remember, if the goal is to have a baby, changing a habit like this is really just a small inconvenience (and only one of many habits you may need to change once you do get pregnant). If you can't totally give up caffeine just yet, maybe have a cup of green tea instead, which is almost certainly better for you than coffee.[9]

Avoid Heavy Metals and Pesticides

Steer away from fish that are more likely to be contaminated with heavy metals[10] since heavy metal accumulation can have an adverse effect on fertility.[11] This is generally a good idea anyway, so perhaps this advice carries even more weight when it comes to the topic of getting and staying pregnant. For starters, skip fish high in mercury like white albacore tuna, grouper, swordfish, king mackerel, shark, swordfish, and tilefish. Instead, you might consider eating low-mercury fish such as pollock, haddock, herring, tilapia, freshwater trout, flounder, and wild salmon. (For a much more complete list, you can go to the National Resources Defense Council's website at www.nrdc.org. You'll be glad to know there are far more items on the "okay to eat" list than there are on the "better stay away" list.) You don't need to avoid eating our seafaring friends entirely; it still seems to be a good idea to consume fish because they are rich in omega-3 fatty acids. Infertile women have been shown to have lower levels of these essential fatty acids.[12] To be on the safer side, supplementation with omega-3 fatty acids is a worthwhile (and mercury-free) choice, especially if you might not be getting enough omega-3 through food. For you fish eaters, it may be encouraging to know that increasing your intake of vitamin C and selenium may help eliminate heavy metals from your system.[13] "Low-mercury" fish are not "no-mercury" fish, so supplement your seafood supper with vitamin C and a multivitamin with selenium. (That goes for him, too!)

Do your best to avoid pesticides and other chemicals, too. (That includes exposure via inhalation, skin contact, or through food.) When it comes to what you eat, be vigilant about washing produce with water *and* soap. Buy organic when possible. One might argue that a small amount of a toxic substance in our food isn't really going to hurt us. Well, it can't possibly help us either! Think of it this way: is it okay if I just add *one drop* of poison to that bowl of minestrone you are about to enjoy? You'd probably prefer that I didn't. It's true that we may not be able to avoid all toxins. However, we can actively purchase and eat foods that don't have added chemicals.

WHAT TO START DOING

There are many natural, drug-free approaches you can try to help reverse infertility. Eating right, exercising, getting enough rest, tracking ovulation, and taking time to "get in the mood" are all on the list.

Focus on a Healthy Diet

Limit your intake of processed, fried, and junk foods, refined sugars, and animal fats[14] like red meat. A diet high in trans fats (those bad

BUT I'M OVER (GASP!) THIRTY!

You wouldn't be the first woman to stress out about getting older and whether you'll be able to get pregnant. Even though fertility is affected by age, it does not mean you are done for once you hit your thirtieth birthday. Yes, it is generally acknowledged that a woman's likelihood of conceiving does decline somewhat in her thirties, and that decline is more marked after thirty-five. And of course we shouldn't rely too much on modern technology to get us knocked up when we are finally darn good and ready. Though there are many factors to consider, I would argue that the healthier you are, the more likely it is that you will be able to achieve a pregnancy. If you do end up seeking fertility treatment, being as healthy as can be still makes a whole lot of sense as you ready your body for a baby.

fats found in junk food)[15] and a high intake of red meat[16] have been linked to an increased risk of endometriosis, a likely cause of infertility. There was a significantly reduced risk for endometriosis in women who had a higher intake of fresh fruits and green vegetables.[17] Avoiding sugar is a good idea as it tends to replace foods you would eat that are far healthier.

Get to Your Optimal Baby-Making Weight

Being really overweight or underweight are both associated with reduced fertility.[18] Eating nutritious food and exercising regularly can help. You don't have to go nuts on the elliptical (too much strenuous exercise can actually have a negative fertility effect), but too many of us aren't getting enough moderate exercise. This is a good reason to ramp it up a bit, especially if you have some pounds to shed. For those folks on the underweight side, gaining a small amount of weight may help your body be more baby-ready.

Try Going Gluten-Free

For some women, avoiding gluten (that stuff commonly found in wheat, rye, and barley products) may help better their chances of getting, and staying, pregnant.[19] It may be worth asking your doctor to screen you for gluten sensitivity or intolerance. It could help explain your unexplained infertility.

Track Ovulation

Know when you are ovulating so you can have sex when you are most fertile. There are handy little urine tests you can take that help you determine just that.

COMING OFF THE PILL?

Women who stop using hormonal contraceptives may have some difficulty getting back to their normal ovulation cycles. Plus, you may have an additional need for certain nutrients. This is all the more reason to make sure you are eating nutritious food and taking your vitamins.

Seek Out Natural Prescription Drug Alternatives

Reexamine those prescription meds you or your partner take. Are they making it more difficult to conceive? Consider looking for natural alternatives.

Have Your Thyroid Function Checked

Low thyroid may also be an undiagnosed reason for infertility.[20] Richard Shames, M.D., and Karilee Shames, R.N., believe "that any man or woman dealing with fertility problems should have the thyroid connection evaluated thoroughly."[21] For information about thyroid trouble and vitamin, mineral, and natural remedies that help

and much more, you may want to read their book *Thyroid Power:*
Ten Steps to Total Health.

Take Time to "Get in the Mood"

Being well-lubricated will help give the little spermies something to
cling too, and the pH (the chemical balance) down there will be more
suited to their survival, too.[22] Plus, being turned on can help you
reach orgasm, which will help move the little guys up your reproductive tract.[23]

Take Time Off, Together

Have you ever heard of those couples that go away on vacation and
bring home an extra little souvenir? Sometimes changing up a stressful life to include a little R&R may be just what your body needs to
conceive. I'm not saying taking a trip to a tropical beach is the answer,
but being stressed is certainly not helping the situation. Along with
eating right, exercising, and taking take your vitamins, taking a
needed break may be a really good idea, whether it results in a pregnancy or not.

Keep Your Relationship Strong

You and your spouse may have already felt some disappointment,
anxiety, worry, and anger over this whole baby situation. This just
isn't easy. There's a lot of pressure here, and the weight of it can strain
your relationship and take away some of the naturalness of being inti-
mate. Forgive the cliché, but Emerson would remind us that life is a
journey, not a destination. It is so important to nurture the relationship first because that exists now, whether or not the future baby-
to-be will. Talk with each other often; express your worries and
concerns. Try to lessen the distance or aloneness you may feel. Talk
about your expectations for parenthood and how important it is to
you. This is a time when it is essential to come together to move
forward, not drift apart. If you do end up pregnant, that comes with

its own slew of new anxieties concerns and life changes. The stronger you are as a couple, the better it will be for the both of you, and the better it will be for baby.

THE VITAMIN AND MINERAL SOLUTION

Antioxidant intake may be a larger part of the infertility puzzle than we think. Current research suggests this could indeed be the case.[24] Though there is much to be said for taking certain individual vitamins, it is important to understand that vitamins tend to work best together. This isn't a magical vitamin cure for infertility; it is an understanding that the body needs to be at its most prepared, baby-ready state in order for pregnancy to occur. Providing your system with essential nutrients only seems smart. Let's give our body the building blocks it needs, so it can best work for us.

Let's start with a good ol' multivitamin. Taking a daily multivitamin is associated with a lower risk of ovulatory infertility.[25] Taking a multivitamin is important while you are pregnant, but it is also important to be taking one before you intend to become pregnant. It helps make up for some of the vitamins you may not be getting in your diet, reduces the risk of having serious birth defects, and may help you get pregnant in the first place!

In one study, women struggling to have a baby for six months to three years showed a significant increase in pregnancy rates when they were supplemented with vitamin E, zinc, selenium, and iron.[26] Other studies have shown that iron[27] may decrease your chances of ovulatory infertility and vitamin C (750 milligrams (mg) per day)[28] may help increase pregnancy rates. Another study found that low concentrations of vitamins E and A were associated with anovulation, the lack of ovulation during a menstrual cycle,[29] suggesting higher levels of these vitamins may be needed to increase fertility potential. Supplementation with multivitamins containing folic acid may improve fertility,[30] as may magnesium (600 mg per day) and selenium (200 micrograms (mcg) per day).[31] Some other specific vitamin dosage suggestions for infertility include 400–1,000 international units (IU) of vitamin E, 15,000 IU of beta-carotene, B_6 (150 mg per day) and a

POLYCYSTIC OVARY SYNDROME

Polycystic ovary syndrome, or PCOS, is an unpleasant condition which has an unpleasant complication of infertility.[33] It is the most common hormonal disorder in women of reproductive age and the most common reason for female infertility,[34] which is kind of a scary thought. With PCOS causing cysts on your ovaries and other symptoms such as irregular periods, acne, dark skin markings, masculine symptoms such as excess body hair (or thinning of hair), decreased breast size, and deepening of one's voice, PCOS can be a real PIA.

It's possible that your doctor will fight PCOS hormone imbalance by suggesting drugs, pills, and surgery that treat symptoms. However, the best approach may be a combination of weight loss and nutrition. If you are carrying excess weight, now may be the best time to resolve to lose it, especially if you have plans to have a family. About half of the gals with PCOS are obese, and women who are overweight are more likely to have the condition.[35] With the growing number of folks who are overweight in this country, we can only imagine that PCOS is a growing problem too. Women with PCOS may also have impaired glucose tolerance, which is a precursor to developing diabetes, another condition influenced by weight gain.

Losing weight (and then maintaining your weight) is easier said than done. However, "[l]osing weight (which can be difficult) has been shown to help with diabetes, high blood pressure, and high cholesterol. Even a weight loss of 5% of total body weight has been shown to help with the imbalance of hormones and also with infertility."[36] Five percent really isn't that much for such a promising return.

Increasing how often you exercise will help reduce stress, and it has the added advantage of weight loss. As for nutrition, embrace a diet that is high in fiber and low in saturated (animal) fats and trans fats.[37] Eat foods with a lower glycemic index, and if you aren't sure what they are, a quick Internet search will bring you plenty of charts and guidelines. For example, foods to avoid contain refined sugars and flours, but this shouldn't be new information. We know reaching for an apple is far better for you than reaching for a donut, even though both contain sugar! As Jack LaLanne's inspiration and mentor, nutritionist Paul Bragg said, "The best part of the donut is the hole." I tend to agree. Additionally, chromium picolinate (200 mcg per day) has been shown to improve glucose tolerance in women with PCOS.[38] Chromium helps level out the highs and lows of blood sugar, but so does exercising and not eating sugar.

You can add additional essential nutrients by supplementing your healthy diet with vitamins A (beta-carotene), C, E, and B-complex, magnesium, selenium, iron, zinc, and omega-3 fatty acids, all of which may help improve fertility.

good B-complex vitamin.[32] It may be more than a little difficult to obtain therapeutic amounts of vitamins and minerals through food. Taking supplements is an inexpensive and easy way to bolster your diet with more of the nutrients you need.

How He Can Help

Seeing as it is just as likely that your man is the reason behind the baby-making blues, there is much to be said for some lifestyle adjustments on his part. There are some simple things your guy can do to help increase your chances of conceiving besides avoiding cigarettes, alcohol, heavy metals, pesticides, and other chemicals. Just like you, he should be focused on eating a really good diet that limits processed, fried, and junk foods, refined sugars, and animal fats,[39] such as red meat. It is also a good idea for your guy to take antioxidant supplements. The data suggest that there isn't necessarily a single vitamin or mineral that will do the trick, but used in combination, the advantages of antioxidant treatment, according to researchers, "cannot be ignored."[40] A recent review of the research done on male infertility and the intake of antioxidants such as vitamin C, E, zinc, selenium, folate (B9), and the carotenoids (vitamin A) showed that in 82 percent of the trials, antioxidant therapy improved either sperm quality or pregnancy rates.[41] Conversely, studies have suggested insufficient levels of antioxidants may contribute to male infertility.[42] Supplementing your man's diet with vitamins and minerals that his body needs anyway is a safe, inexpensive, and potentially effective way to increase the chances that his sperm will be able to shine when the time is right. He can also help ensure his best sperm count by keeping "the boys" cool. Wearing boxers instead of "tighty whities" will

PELVIC INFLAMMATORY DISEASE (PID)

Another nasty little problem that can be the reason behind infertility is pelvic inflammatory disease, which is an inflammation or infection of your reproductive organs. Scar tissue can form and block pathways for reproduction, and PID increases the risk of tubal pregnancy, which is why infertility is a likely consequence of the disease. You might notice symptoms such as pain in your abdomen, pain during sex, a fever, and/or unusual vaginal discharge; it may be painful to pee and/or you might experience irregular menstrual bleeding. Douching, intrauterine devices (IUDs), and multiple sex partners may increase your risk for PID. Most often, these infections are acquired after getting an STD like chlamydia or gonorrhea, but you can also get PID after a miscarriage, abortion, or childbirth. If your physician thinks you have PID, he or she will probably give you antibiotics, but unfortunately, this won't reverse damage that may already be done.[43] Prevention is the best medicine, but if you've got it, it is best to get rid of it as soon as possible to prevent further damage and potential infertility. And while you are at it, take appropriate measures to boost your immune system. Eat yogurt to help replenish good bacteria when taking antibiotics. Take immune boosters like vitamins C, E, A, and the B vitamins. A multivitamin with zinc should also be on your list. For more information about the role of vitamins and infection and immunity, look into the chapter on urinary tract infections (UTIs), which goes into more detail about these nutrients and their importance.

provide a more sperm-friendly environment. Keeping out of steaming hot tubs or saunas will also keep his sperm count higher.

VITAMINS, MINERALS, AND MISCARRIAGE

There is no comfort to be found in words when a baby dies, and I'm not about to try. It is truly an awful experience to have. Though it may not seem like the same thing, miscarriage is considered to be another part of the definition of infertility: the inability to carry a pregnancy to full term.[44] Though we may not know what causes a miscarriage, we do know that nutrition may help prevent them.

There are all sorts of things that could account for a miscarriage; nutrition is just one possible piece of the puzzle. There is a link between a diet low in antioxidants and recurrent pregnancy loss.[45] Consider that even if you feel you are eating well and taking care of yourself, you may still not be getting enough of the antioxidants such as vitamin E, vitamin C, beta-carotene, zinc, and selenium. As many as 50 to 60 percent of recurrent miscarriages may be attributed to oxidative stress,[46] indicating that for some women, a higher intake of antioxidants may be needed. Research has shown that women who have experienced recurrent miscarriages have significantly lower levels of antioxidants (like vitamins C and E) than healthy women.[47] Another link is that women with high levels of homocysteine are more likely to experience recurrent miscarriages.[48] Higher levels of homocysteine in the blood are caused by deficiencies in certain nutrients like B vitamins (B_6, B_{12}, and folic acid) suggesting that B vitamin supplementation could be helpful.[49]

Everything outlined in this chapter to help better understand certain risks for infertility and what can be done about them also applies to miscarriage. You got pregnant, now we need to find out how you might better be able to stay that way.

None of this suggests that there is something you could have done to prevent a miscarriage. In most cases, there's nothing you did or could have done to stop it from happening. I hope you take from this section some comfort in the idea that there may be a nutritional connection. If that happens to be true for you, this is only good news.

GETTING YOUR BODY READY FOR BABY: YOUR NUTRIENT CHECKLIST

Vitamins work well together, so take them together. You can always start small and then ramp up your dosage to your optimal amount.

B-complex: Take twice a day. Look for 25–50 mg each of B_1, B_2, B_3, and B_6 and 400 mcg of folic acid (B_9); the amounts of B_{12}, biotin, and pantothenic acid can vary. Consider taking additional B_6 (to get 150 mg per day) in addition to the amounts present in your B-complex.

Vitamin A: A powerful antioxidant, take 5,000–15,000 IU per day in the form of beta-carotene; or drink all you want of fresh, raw carrot juice; or eat other foods rich in beta-carotene, like sweet potatoes, pumpkin, and green leafy veggies.

Vitamin C: 6,000–18,000 mg per day; take more or less as desired.

Vitamin E: 400–1,000 IU per day in the form of mixed tocopherols (best) or d-alpha tocopherol; take separately from your iron supplement.

Iron: In the form of ferrous fumarate, ferrous gluconate, or carbonyl iron, take 18–27 mg per day; take separately from your vitamin E and calcium supplements.

Magnesium: In the form of citrate or gluconate, take 600 mg per day.

Omega-3 fatty acids: Look for a fish oil supplement that contains 900–1,000 mg total of EPA and DHA omega-3 fatty acids. Be sure to read the label. A tablet that contains 1,000 mg of fish oil may only contain 300 mg of omega-3 fatty acids. You will want to take three of those a day to get the optimum dose.

Selenium: 100–200 mcg a day.

Chromium: To help improve glucose tolerance, take 200 mcg per day.

Multivitamin: Take twice a day. Look for one that also contains 15–30 mg of zinc.

RECOMMENDED READING

Shames, R. L., K. H. Shames. *Thyroid Power: Ten Steps to Total Health*. New York, NY: HarperResource, 2001.

Brighthope, I. *The Vitamin Cure for Diabetes*. Laguna Beach, CA: Basic Health Publications, 2012.

CHAPTER 10

SEX DRIVE: WAIT . . . WHAT?

"I admit, I have a tremendous sex drive.
My boyfriend lives forty miles away."
—PHYLLIS DILLER

If you don't have it, you know it. And the love of your life probably knows it too. It sure is hard to hide something that usually requires someone else's involvement.

How often, say, during these last few weeks has it been late in the evening and you are craving quality time with your pillow, but you gaze at your sweetheart and wonder, when was the last time you had the energy for a little mattress mambo? Lately, you have felt so exhausted, you couldn't manage turning the dial on the dishwater to "on," let alone be turned on yourself. If it just wasn't so much work taking off clothes . . .

Wait a second. How unfair is *that*? We put all our time and energy into taking care of all these important things that have-to-get-done-now, and we end up not having the energy or desire for something we actually can enjoy. Yes, *enjoy*. Have we forgotten? Has it been that long?

WHAT'S UP?

Before we go find something else to do for fun, let's take a look at some common reasons why it may be hard to get in the mood. For women, sexual desire is emotional and physical. We can't just pop a pill and be ready to go. We have to be physically ready and in the right state of mind, too. For instance, if you are suffering through a crappy relationship or are dealing with abuse, you aren't going to be in the right state of mind to get down and dirty. The way you feel about yourself—your body image—also plays into your sexuality. If you feel unsexy, it's likely that you won't want sex! Sometimes it's hard to feel attractive when this country paints such an unrealistic image of the perfect girl, and last time you checked the mirror, you weren't her. But there are so many women out there who *are* in happy relationships and they don't look like "her" either, so give yourself a break. If you aren't happy with your body, and there's a good health-conscious, confidence-boosting, mood-enhancing reason to make a change, do it! But if your idea of "fixing" yourself comes with a massive plastic surgery bill and a desire turn your body into someone else's, you need to stop and take the time to find out why. What makes you awesome, *as is*? There are people on this planet that love you just the way you are. Why can't you be one of them?

THE SEX DRIVE STOPPERS

Loss of sex drive is a symptom, not a disease. It merely highlights that perhaps there is something else causing a change in your sexual appetite. There are probably dozens of things that could affect your wanting, or not wanting, to have sex.

Stress

Life isn't always easy (is it ever?) but if you are anxious, over-worked or stressed, it is *really* hard to get excited about sex. Can you remember the last time you were on vacation? Did you happen to notice anything about your sex drive? Perhaps it is just the intoxicating air of the tropics that lured you into a passionate sex-capade that week, or maybe it was something else: stress-free time with the one you love. It's no surprise that your libido was excited about a vacation too. And yet, life doesn't allow for continual carefree retreats to a Caribbean paradise. With work, family, and everything else we pack onto our to-do list, it doesn't always accommodate for extended breaks, and neither does our bank account.

However, that's no excuse for not taking a little "you" time here and there to buffer a busy week's schedule. Sadly, stress is just a part of life, but if it is interfering with the things you like to do (like, um, sex?), then perhaps it is time to reevaluate what steps you can take to lessen the strain on your system so you feel more like leaping into the sack with your doe-eyed hubby. Seek out stress-reducing activities like exercise, yoga, meditation, and massage. Trim down your schedule where you can and insert time for activities you like to do instead, even sex! Take some deep breaths. Laugh. Limit mood-altering substances (like caffeine, sugar, and alcohol) that may make you feel nice for a while, but then bring you crashing down hard.

Depression

If you feel down and lack interest in the things you once liked to do, it isn't surprising that sex ends up on the "not interested" list. Take some time to read through the chapter on stress, anxiety, and depression for even more natural treatment advice.

Illness and Infection

If things aren't operating up to standard down below, it's not likely that you are going to want to have sex. Perhaps sex is painful, uncomfortable, and not enjoyable. If sickness is behind your choice to wear your "do not cross zone" panties, then this can certainly be addressed. Have your doctor help you understand what is going on (whether it's illness down there or elsewhere) so you can take the steps you need to get back to 100 percent. Your health should come first, and feeling better can only help when it comes to sex.

Aging and Other Life Changes

All right. Supposedly, getting older doesn't help since it is hypothesized that as ovulation becomes more infrequent and eventually ceases, so does our sexual appetite. Perhaps it seems only natural that as our body becomes less able to reproduce that it would also have less desire to attempt to do so. Perhaps that super sex-crazed feeling we used to notice during ovulation is just not there as it was. Is lowered sex drive just a natural response in a body that no longer will bear children? Before we go shrugging our shoulders and picking up a new pastime (golf, anyone?), there are plenty of women out there that are having the best sex of their lives even during menopausal transitions.

Other thoughts on lack of libido suggest that the hormone imbalance many women experience during menopausal transitions (and postpartum for that matter) wreak all sorts of havoc on us physically and affect our feelings about sex. It's hard to be interested in doing it if you are tired, moody, and lacking energy. Speaking of hormones, estrogen loss is thought to be a culprit in decreased sexual interest. Estrogen keeps our girl parts moist and plump; lack of estrogen as experienced while aging can cause the vaginal area to be dry and irritated and make us not want to put anything penis-shaped in there. Testosterone—yes, testosterone—also decreases as we age, and this may make us not as interested in sex. This does not mean you need to load your body up with potentially dangerous hormonal drugs to modify your hormone levels. Diet, exercise, and nutritional supplements can help instead, safely and naturally. For more information, read the chapter in this book on menopause.

Relationships

It takes two to tango, as it were, so we can't forget about the other important part of the sex equation: that person you head off to bed with. Good or bad, your relationship determines the amount of sex you will have to a very significant degree. He may not be banging down your door to drag you to the bedroom, and that may be part of the issue. Sometimes, a rocky relationship can get in the way of wanting to make love. Maybe your idea of lovemaking doesn't fit his idea of lovemaking. Maybe you operate on different schedules or have tremendous responsibilities that keep you from each other's arms. Or you may have a spectacular, loving relationship, but there's just not the time or the energy for sex. And the list goes on.

There are hundreds of books on sex and relationships, and I'll leave it to you to do a little research about what would work best for you and yours. Take time together to read about what you both can do to ignite that flame. If you know that somehow your relationship situation is behind your no-sex status quo, you owe it to yourself (and he to himself) to address this. Sometimes, relationship counseling can help set the stage for just such a discussion. It is easy to let this part of the relationship slide; romance takes effort. You may have to really work at making sex a priority.

THE SEX DRIVE STARTERS

Staying as healthy as possible is probably one of the best ways to naturally boost your desire. It should not come as a shock that eating right, exercising, and getting enough rest is important. Don't underestimate the power of any of this. Feeling your best will make you more likely to want to get into the mood.

Exercise

Take a walk. Go work in the garden. Crank up your favorite tunes and dance your heart out in the living room. Go for a swim. Go on a bike ride. Break out those dusty DVDs and do some yoga or that cardio workout you've been meaning to try. Set a goal by signing up for a local race or charity event that will motivate you to get running, biking, or swimming. Get a friend to do it with you. When it comes down to it, just *move*. You will manage stress better if you stay active, and you will reduce the likelihood that you'll get any number of chronic illnesses, and yes, it can also increase your sex drive.

Rest

If you aren't well-rested, it is hard find the energy to have sex. But, sometimes, sex is outweighed by the desire to get more rest. Hmm. Have sex . . . or sleep. I'm sure there's been more than a few times where sleep wins, hands down. But maybe you can accomplish both.

Must we rob Peter to pay Paul? Or can life be modified in such a way that you have time to sleep *and* time to play?

Nutrition

The better you eat, the better you'll feel. Take care of yourself, starting with what you eat and drink. Eat organic, nourishing, whole foods. Get more veggies onto your plate and less red meat. Start drinking fresh, raw vegetable juice. Limit sugar, caffeine and alcohol. Oh, and take your vitamins!

KEEPING UP HIS END OF THE BARGAIN

A good diet with extra zinc and vitamin C are important to male fertility. He should eat healthy meals and limit his intake of refined and processed foods, fast foods, and animal fats, and avoid foods containing nitrates (such as red hot dogs and deli meats). Smoking and alcohol use don't help keep his man bits interested in lovemaking either. Just as with us, stress, depression, and lack of exercise or rest can also dampen his drive.

Vitamins and Minerals

There are vitamins and minerals you can add to your diet that naturally help balance hormones, manage stress, fight fatigue and lack of energy, and improve mood. This doesn't mean that a vitamin is necessarily going to make you want to bound off to the bedroom this very second, but if a safe, natural supplement helps you feel better, it may indeed have that result.

Extra vitamin C may be just the thing to take if you want to increase how often you have sex and also improve your mood.[1] A dose of 3,000 milligrams (mg) per day of vitamin C was shown to do just that in a randomized, double-blind, placebo-controlled study.[2] The vitamin C group had sex more often than the placebo group and the vitamin C takers showed a decrease in Beck Depression Inventory (BDI) scores. (The BDI is a depression questionnaire with a scoring scale.) The authors mentioned that vitamin C "modulates catecholaminergic activity, decreases stress reactivity, approach anxiety and prolactin release, improves vascular function, and increases oxytocin release. These processes are relevant to sexual behavior and mood."[3] That's a lot of fancy scientific talk, but it boils down to "get busy more often and feel better." That's not bad for just a few cents for a few C tablets each day.

Being tired and moody isn't much of a turn-on for either partner. Fortunately, the B vitamins are useful for bettering your mood and increasing energy. Low levels of folate (B_9) and B_{12} have been noted in folks with depression,[4] suggesting supplementation could be beneficial, and B vitamins help fight fatigue, too.[5] Vitamin D can help you feel less down,[6] making it more likely you'll be up for some lovin'. Iron can help, too. A number of us are deficient in iron,[7] the most common symptom of which is feeling tired.[8] Iron may help reduce fatigue[9], especially for those of us who are losing some every month during our periods.

Sometimes, physical discomfort can put sexual desire on the back burner. Perhaps you don't have an infection but you still feel irritated, dry, or sore down there. Spread on pure, natural vitamin E to help soothe and heal sensitive skin.

DO WHAT WORKS

It's okay to desire more physical interaction with your honey. It's also okay not to! We aren't machines, for goodness sake. Intimacy is more than just a frolic beneath the sheets. Don't let any perceived pressure put you in a spot where you think that you have to be putting out in order to meet some sort of outside expectation. That being said, if you wish to have a more active sex life, take the time to sort out what really might be getting in the way. Is there a physical reason? An emotional reason? Keep reading, keep learning, and keep communicating with your partner. Take care of yourself. Take care of each other. Do what feels right and natural for you both.

CHAPTER 11

MENOPAUSE: BEFORE, DURING, AND AFTER

"I know God will not give me anything I can't handle.
I just wish that He didn't trust me so much."
—MOTHER TERESA

Finally! A permanent vacation from your period! Yay! Some of us have been really looking forward to this.

To signify "becoming a woman" oh-so-many years ago, my parents took me out for my favorite Chinese dinner. I'd be lying if I said the reason for our dinner didn't put a bit of a damper on the occasion (we're celebrating this?!) but I ordered my favorite dish, "Bean Curd Family Style," and ate my fill of tofu in relative silence, appreciative of a tasty dinner away from our sugar-free, homegrown organic garden, raw-veggie-juice-centric vegetarian kitchen.

I never did ask what the prize was for making it to menopause. (More tofu?)

WHAT WE CAN EXPECT

Some of us have been itching to get rid of our monthly visitor for a while. It has been a royal pain in the keister for decades, after all. However, losing one annoying thing about being a woman is replaced now by a list of other annoying things as we venture into menopause. First of all, for many of us, menstruation won't just stop. It will just happen when our bodies feel like it, causing a pretty irregular (and inconvenient) schedule for a year or three. Then there are all the other lovely little symptoms we may have to experience during this transition: hot flashes, sweating, and sleeping issues are very common. We may also experience vaginal atrophy and dryness; memory issues; headaches; mood swings—up, down, and all around; bloating; weight gain; fatigue; cramps; vaginal infections; achy joints; hair loss (or hair gained where we least want it); less interest in sex; a pounding or palpitating heart; and urinary incontinence.[1] How nice. Once our period is gone for good our menopausal symptoms may ease up, but now we are at a higher risk for dangers like heart disease and osteoporosis.

Sigh.

Is it ever *not* difficult to be a woman?

IN THE DOCTOR'S HANDBAG: HRT

If we take a look around our doctor's medicine bag, it's probably filled with hormones, and that's about it. Menopause has kind of been turned into a disease by the medical community—which it isn't—and drug therapy has been their response to the "problem."

Hormone replacement therapy (HRT) is pretty scary. "Several major studies have questioned the health benefits and risks of hormone replacement therapy, including the risk of developing breast cancer, heart attacks, strokes, and blood clots."[2] There can also be an increased risk for heart disease (for older women), gallbladder disease, endometrial cancer, and uterine cancer.[3] HRT has been evaluated as a drug treatment whose "overall health risks exceeded benefits."[4] That was the conclusion of a particular study of over 16,500 postmenopausal women, originally intended to span 8.5 years. It was canceled more than three years sooner because too many women were getting invasive breast cancer.[5] Combine the risk of these life-threatening diseases with unpleasant side effects like bloating, sore breasts, headaches, mood swings, irregular bleeding, and nausea,[6] and HRT just doesn't seem worth it, and many women who have tried it would agree.[7]

Well, there is some good news. One study concluded that when it came to breast cancer, ladies who used HRT (as opposed to those who didn't) had "more favorable tumors."[8]

"Favorable tumors." Really?

"Don't worry, Mrs. Smith. You have good cancer!"

"That's a relief, doc. I mean, it could have been bad cancer!"

We have to ask: if hormone replacement therapy is the reason we have a cancerous lump in the first place, is a "more favorable tumor" really a triumph of modern medicine?

The main reason we gals turn to HRT is to get some relief from undesirable menopausal symptoms. However, trading one discomfort for another (and increasing the chance that we'll get cancer and then die, or get some other horrid disease . . . then die) may be why so many women are saying no to HRT.

There is much you can do to ease your menopausal symptoms safely and naturally, reducing the likelihood that you'll feel the need to turn to hormone therapy for relief. Not to put too fine a point on it, but even if natural alternatives *don't* work for you, they're still a heck of a lot safer to try out. If they do the trick, it's a win-win situation.

THIS SOUNDS AN AWFUL LOT LIKE PMS

It's hard to ignore that many of the undesirable symptoms of menopause also happen to be familiar to those of us who had premenstrual syndrome (PMS) or have suffered physically from stress: headaches, sleeping problems, mood swings, fatigue, bloating, cramps . . . maybe we thought that when our period was almost over, this stuff would be over, too. Well, not yet. Those crazy little hormones are still at work. And stress? Well, at least *some* stress sure seems unavoidable. Fear not! Balancing hormones is a key part of managing menopause, and nutrition and lifestyle can do oodles to help.

Mood Changes

If your moods are swinging, there's a lot you can do naturally to get them evened out. The PMS chapter in this book, as well as the chapter on stress, anxiety, and depression, gives numerous nutritional recommendations for how to balance our emotions.

Trouble Sleeping and Fatigue

For help with those restless nights and exhaustion-filled days, read the sections on insomnia and fatigue in the chapters on stress, anxiety, and depression and on PMS.

Cramps

Menstrual cramps are Mother Nature's punch to the gut. If menopause is still bringing on the cramps (or maybe, in your case, Mother Nature has just waited until now to get feisty), read about how to punch back in the PMS chapter. The very nutrients you needed to help curtail cramps then are the nutrients you need to do the same now.

Headaches

Who needs 'em? If you are ready to minimize the number of these puppies you get, read the sections on headaches in the chapters on PMS and on stress, anxiety, and depression.

Bloating

The nutritional recommendation for bloating and PMS are going to come in handy for menopause, too. If you want the water to stay "out", then you'll want to keep from putting salt "in." All that extra sodium is going to influence water retention. As for vitamins, B_6 is your friend: 100–300 milligrams (mg) a day.[9] Take it along with a B-complex vitamin, which will probably have a measure of B_6 in it, too. In PMS, just 200 mg per day of magnesium helped reduce weight gain, bloating, and swelling of hands and legs.[10] For menopause, you may wish to take much more than that; 1,000 mg per day.[11] A similar dose of calcium, 1,000–1,200 mg per day, was also an effective water retention reducer in PMS,[12] and as far as I'm concerned, that's a good reason to give it a try for menopause, our other hormonal adversary.

WHAT TO STOP DOING

The advice for good health that has always been true continues to be true: stop smoking and avoid sugar, red meat, caffeine, and alcohol. Of course, we aren't dead yet, and it's no fun to feel like we are prematurely acting that way. For some of us, simply limiting our bad habits to a very occasional event is more reasonable, especially if we are handling things well—except when it comes to smoking. There isn't a "reasonable" amount to smoke. That just needs to stop.

AGING

"The idea is to die young as late as possible."
—ASHLEY MONTAGU

The best plan for looking and feeling great later is taking care of yourself now. The advice for aging well doesn't really change much from the advice for staying healthy and attractive at a younger age: Eat right. Exercise. Don't smoke. Stay out of tanning booths and excessive amounts of sun. Smile. And take your vitamins. If you want to add "buy lots of expensive wrinkle creams," that's fine, too. Goodness knows, we are using them anyway.

WHAT TO START DOING, OR KEEP DOING

Here's the big one: we must reduce stress. Stress makes menopause a whole lot worse, and if you want to feel better, stress reduction is the first thing to tackle. It's always a good idea to exercise (it will help keep muscle tone and limit weight gain); eat small, regular, nourishing meals; and keep doctor's appointments for regular checkups of cholesterol levels, blood pressure, and breast exams (to name a few). We'll also need to keep an eye on getting extra nutrients to help prevent osteoporosis and heart disease.

MANAGING MENOPAUSE WITH VITAMINS AND NUTRITION

Let's take a closer look at what nutrition can do for some of the common symptoms of menopause like hot flashes, vaginal atrophy, urinary urgency, memory loss, and, unfortunately, more.

Hot Flashes

We can shed layers of clothing, ban flannel sheets, and open windows on frigid days, but we can also manage hot flashes with diet. It appears that estrogen decreases in menopause, but phytoestrogens, substances found in plants that have estrogen-like effects, can be added into the diet to compensate for their loss. Even though the results are mixed, several studies have shown that soy may be especially helpful for reducing the frequency, severity, and/or duration of hot flashes. After sixteen weeks of treatment with soy isoflavone extract, over 60 percent of women in one study reduced the number of hot flashes they had each day.[13] Another trial showed that soy isoflavone extract helped women experienced a decrease in the incidence and severity of hot flashes in as few as two weeks.[14] Another demonstrated that after twelve weeks of treatment with soy protein isolate powder, nearly half of the women reduced the number of daily hot flashes.[15] Increasing our consumption of foods rich in phytoestrogens (namely soy products) is worth a try. This means that tofu is our friend (and not just a coveted ingredient in my menarche celebration Chinese din-din) as we venture into menopause, as are other food sources of phytoestrogens like flaxseed (that's a potent one!), sesame seeds, garlic, beans, chickpeas, lentils, dried apricots, whole grains, prunes, and alfalfa, to name just a few. If you get gassy and bloated form eating too much soy, consider eating fermented soy instead (like miso or tempeh), which is easier to digest.[16]

James Balch, M.D., and Phyllis Balch, C.N.C., state, "Dairy products, sugar, and meat cause most hot flashes"[17] so it's best that you limit your consumption to some yogurt, and fish rather than red meat. Additionally, they recommend that you take vitamin E, starting with 400 international units (IU) and gradually (I would say over a period of weeks) increasing your dose (up to 1,600 IU) until hot flashes cease.[18] Vitamin C, 3,000–10,000 mg per day, is also recommended for hot flashes, as is taking a B-complex several times a day.[19] Keep an eye on potassium, too. If your hot flashes are severe, you'll want to get much more of this nutrient into your diet. Beans, lentils, peas, spinach, oranges, bananas, strawberries, prunes, raisins, potatoes, and avocados pack a potassium punch (and many contain those helpful phytoestrogens, too). For those of you wishing to reduce the size of that pool of sweat you woke up in last night, potassium may help control all that icky, excessive perspiration.[20]

Vaginal Atrophy

I guess the menopausal symptom of "vaginal atrophy" is a nicer way of labeling what we might call a dried-out and shrinking vagina. Continuing to have sex will help keep this from becoming a problem. (To put it bluntly, it's kind of a "use it or lose it" situation.) But if we are starting to feel uncomfortable down there, no matter how much action that area is or is not getting, a few things may help. Using lubrication is a good idea, and we also shouldn't underestimate the importance of being turned on before we have at it. If you feel sore or itchy, break open a vitamin E capsule and spread it over the afflicted area for relief. Continue to take oral vitamin E supplements, too: 400–800 international units (IU) a day.[21] Oral vitamin D may also be helpful.[22]

"I Have to Pee. Again."

As our lady bits get a bit dried out, a common side effect is the need to scope every restaurant, store, or house for a bathroom before we even get down to eating, shopping, or visiting. Limiting our caffeine and alcohol intake can help, as can shedding excess pounds. Higher intakes of vitamin D may be preventative,[23] as may increased potassium intake, B_6 and niacin.[24] For that "oops" leakage that happens when we laugh, sneeze, or exercise, kegels (that secret little pelvic floor exercise) can strengthen the muscles we use to keep from letting our bladder drain at will.[25]

Infections "Down There"

You may be uncomfortable because of some unwanted visitors. Yeast or other nasty little bacterium can cause intense irritation. If you are itchy, sore, red, swollen or just otherwise uncomfortable in the nether region, read the chapters on yeast infections and bacterial vaginosis to see if they may be behind your distress. If a urinary tract infection is to blame, there's a chapter on that, too.

Heart Palpitations

If you are attached at the lip to your coffee cup, now's a great time to change that relationship and eliminate caffeine as the reason behind your acrobatic ticker. You may also need more magnesium. Match your magnesium intake with your calcium intake; we tend to get far more of the latter than the former. Carolyn Dean, M.D., N.D., states, "We take far too much calcium compared to magnesium, mostly because we've been told calcium is the most important mineral for bone health, but magnesium is just as crucial for bone and heart health."[26]

Memory Loss

If you want to help boost your ability to think clearly and remember where you put your keys . . . and better yet, where you parked your car . . . lecithin may be just the thing to try. The B vitamins are very important for normal brain function, especially choline (considered to be a part of the B group).[27] Choline is an essential nutrient, one that has been shown to improve brain function in animal studies.[28] Choline given to pregnant rats improved the memory of their babies, and this remained the case even when the little ones were elderly.[29] "When rat pups received choline supplements (*in utero* or during the second week of life), their brain function changed, resulting in the lifelong memory enhancement."[30] Pretty cool, huh? Maybe our mothers didn't load up on lecithin when we were in the womb, so now's our chance.

Choline can be found in lecithin as part of phosphatidyl choline.

Lecithin is a product derived from soy, available in granular form (best) or tablet form (okay—but you have to take about eight to ten of them to get the same dose that's present in a spoonful of granules). Granules provide a kick-butt 1,700 mg or so of phosphatidyl choline in each tablespoon, along with other good-for-you nutrients like 1,000 mg of phosphatidyl inositol and 2,200 mg of essential fatty acids. Mix some into yogurt or a fruit smoothie. I prefer to pour a dry spoonful into my mouth followed by a few swallows of water to avoid having to chew the stuff. Lecithin is an emulsifier that helps our body absorb fat-soluble vitamins like vitamin E; it also helps keep cholesterol from becoming a problem, helps prevent arteriosclerosis, aids in the absorption of vitamin A and thiamine (B_1), and is protective against cardiovascular disease,[31] all great reasons to remember to take it!

Zinc and iron also help improve memory. One study showed that after eight weeks of supplementation with 30 mg of zinc, 30 mg of iron, or both, the short-term memory of women improved by 15–20 percent.[32]

Stiff, Painful, and Aching Joints

Margie is a very active fifty-six-year-old working gal. It was more than a little disconcerting when she was finding herself unable to fully close her hands or kneel down without pain, let alone get back up comfortably. Joint dysfunction may be just another symptom of nutrient deficiency, and in Margie's case, that's exactly what was going on. Niacinamide (500 mg per day) completely resolved this issue. Back in the 1950s, William Kaufman, M.D., was successfully treating joint dysfunction with niacinamide in doses anywhere from 400–2,250 mg per day.[33] If you want to give it a go, start taking 100–150 mg of niacinamide at each meal and gradually raise your dose until your symptoms go away. You could also chop a larger tablet into sections, and take that in divided doses. The goal is to get rid of the aches and pains without bringing on any nausea, a possible side effect of too much niacinamide. Find the balanced dose that works for you. Your bendy parts will thank you!

Hair Loss

Losing your locks? Male-pattern baldness isn't just for men. (Darn it, anyway!) Unfortunately, there are quite a few factors that can cause us ladies to lose our hair. Vitamin deficiency, iron deficiency, hormonal changes, thyroid disease, diabetes, and poor diet are just some of the reasons our tresses might be thinning. Thank goodness vitamins may help improve the health and growth of our hair. (And in the right places!) Generous quantities of vitamin C (3,000–10,000 mg per day), the B vitamins, (notably pantothenic acid (B$_5$) 300 mg per day, pyridoxine (B$_6$) 150 mg per day, and niacin (B$_3$) 150 mg per day), and vitamin E (400–1,000 IU daily) are recommended for hair loss.[34] Zinc and a touch of copper (to improve immune function and encourage hair growth), omega fatty acids (to improve dry, brittle hair),[35] and magnesium (for stress)[36] may also be helpful.

If your hair isn't sticking to your head, it's time to focus on diet and de-stressing. Dr. Dean explains, "As stress hormones are revved up in the adrenal glands, that action also triggers the production of more male hormones. A diet high in refined carbohydrates and excess body fat only makes things worse by further stimulating hormone production."[37] Take a moment to glance over the helpful nutrients your stressed self needs in the chapter on stress, anxiety, and depression.

Managing Weight Gain

It's no surprise that exercise is on the to-do list. It has always been helpful for shedding those pesky ounces. It will make us feel better, think better, sleep better, and even help our sex drive. It's harder to lose excess pounds as we get older, making it all that more important that we exercise (and do so every day) *and* eat a good diet. Maybe there is truly a magic weight loss pill out there somewhere—one that won't just kill us, caffeinate us, or clean out our wallets. So far, I'm not impressed with what is available. Anyway, some pills say they are most effective when combined with diet and exercise. Hmm. Perhaps we can just remove the middle man.

No matter what pill we are swallowing, what we eat day in and day out and what we do physically day in and day out will be a far better indicator of whether we will reach and maintain our weight goal. Moderate, regular, and varied aerobic exercise including weight training, combined with a high-fiber, raw-food rich, low sugar, low salt, low to no alcohol, whole-grain, diet, together with healthy fats (not saturated or trans fats), and vegetarian-based protein (and a whole lot less red meat) is what gets the job done. Cut back a bit on your calorie intake. Don't stuff yourself; don't starve yourself either. To help manage spikes and drops in blood sugar that send us straight to the chips in the cupboard, take 200–400 micrograms (mcg) per day of chromium picolinate. Chromium won't get rid of hunger; it's not a diet pill. It does not exert any kind of mind control over subjects who choose to use it. Evening out highs and lows in blood sugar may help us control our own impulses instead of succumbing to the will of the midafternoon sugar fest.

None of this is a secret. It just isn't easy. If you want to manage your weight, feel better from head to toe, and prevent disease, the solution stays the same, and it takes effort every day. I wish I could say, "Just take this vitamin and you'll be all set!" It just doesn't work that way. We can't eat like angels every meal and exercise like Olympic champions every day, but a majority of what we put in our bodies and do with our bodies should be focused on a achieving a healthier self.

Digestive Trouble

Do you get that uncomfortable, heavy stomach sensation after eating a meal? You may not have overeaten, but you feel as if there's a bunch of rocks in your belly and you anticipate a night of gas, bloating, acid reflux, burping, and discomfort, all symptoms that can go along with a poorly digested meal. (The protein-based, carbohydrate-packed, fat-laden meals at our local barbecue joint do it to me every time!) As we age, we may notice that our digestion isn't what it used to be. Digestive enzymes can help.

Raw food naturally contains enzymes that aid digestion. When we cook our food, those enzymes are destroyed. This makes it that much harder for our bodies to break down what we eat and get the most nutrition out of it. Having our cooked food along with raw food (aim for 50 percent of the meal) is a way to get those beneficial enzymes into our diet, but this isn't always possible, especially if we are out and about. If you want to reduce unpleasant gastrointestinal symptoms, you may want to try taking digestive enzyme supplements. (I carry them in my purse!) Pancreatin (an animal source of enzymes) is made up of amylase, protease, and lipase—enzymes that digest carbohydrates, protein, and fat respectively. You can also obtain vegetarian, plant-based enzyme supplements. Take these after one of those gut-busting meals, and you may find you spare yourself some digestive despair.

Osteoporosis

There is a lot we can do with nutrition to prevent osteoporosis. Not smoking, limiting sugar and animal fats, and avoiding caffeine, alcohol, and soda pop are all good ideas, as they were earlier in our lives and still are now. Exercise helps build bone, so staying active is a must. Vitamins and minerals help too, as certain deficiencies increase your risk of osteoporosis.

We hear an awful lot about calcium, and yes, it is very important to make sure you get adequate amounts. It's most beneficial to get enough calcium (along with vitamin D, which is necessary for calcium absorption) when you are a young woman, well before menopause, but calcium-rich diets and calcium and vitamin D can still build bone mass in later years.[38] You may want to supplement your calcium intake with 1,000–2,000 IU of vitamin D a day, especially if you aren't exposed to much sunshine. Magnesium should be taken with calcium, in similar amounts. Along with 1,000–1,500 mg per day of calcium, it's recommended that you get 800–1,000 mg per day of magnesium.[39] Other important bone nutrients include vitamin C, vitamins B_6, B_{12}, and folic acid, manganese, zinc, and copper. Boron improves calcium absorption. Fruits, vegetables, and nuts are good sources of boron, and you may also find that your calcium supplement includes some.

MANAGING MENOPAUSE WITH NUTRIENTS

Below are a number of nutrients that boost immunity, fight symptoms of menopause, and are protective against osteoporosis and heart disease.

Vitamin A: An immunity booster, take 25,000 IU per day in the form of beta-carotene.

B-complex: Take one twice a day that includes 25–50 mg each of B_1, B_2, B_3, and B_6, 400 mcg of folic acid, 50 mcg of B_{12}, and 50 mg of pantothenic acid (or more when under stress).

Vitamin B_3: When needed, take an additional 50–500 mg of nicotinic acid; or try 500–1,000 mg of "flush-free" (inositol hexaniacinate) niacin; or take 100–500 mg of niacinamide. Note that these are "as needed" amounts, so your total daily dose may be higher or lower depending on your symptoms.

Vitamin B_6: When needed, take an additional 50–200 mg per day.

Calcium: In the form of carbonate or citrate, take 1,000–2,000 mg a day with vitamin D; take calcium separately from your iron supplement.

Chromium: In the form of chromium picolinate, take 200–400 mcg a day.

Vitamin C: 6,000–18,000 mg per day; take more or less as needed.

Vitamin E: 400–1,600 IU per day in the form of mixed tocopherols or d-alpha tocopherol; take separately from your iron supplement.

Vitamin D: 1,000–2,000 IU per day, along with calcium.

Iron: In the form of ferrous fumarate, ferrous gluconate or carbonyl iron, take 18 mg per day; take separately from your vitamin E and calcium supplements.

Magnesium: In the form of citrate or gluconate, take 600–1,000 mg per day.

Omega-3 fatty acids: Look for a fish oil supplement that contains 900–1,000 mg total of EPA and DHA omega-3 fatty acids. A tablet that contains 1,000 mg of fish oil may only contain 300 mg of omega-3 fatty acids. You will want to take three of those a day to get the optimum dose.

Copper: 2 mg per day.

Selenium: 100–200 mcg per day.

Multivitamin: Take twice daily. Look for one that contains manganese (2–4 mg) and 15–30 mg of zinc.

Lecithin: Take one tablespoon daily in the form of granules.

Digestive enzymes: Take with meals to aid digestion.

Heart Disease

It's the single leading cause of death for women in the United States.[40] Don't let yourself become a statistic. Read about lifestyle modifications and the importance of vitamins and nutrition for the prevention of heart disease in the chapter on stress, anxiety, and depression.

Making the Most of Menopause

All right, so maybe no one is going to throw us a parade for making it to or through menopause. Still, let's have our own internal party (whoo hoo!) with the knowledge that we are doing all we can to make these years as healthy and productive as all the years we've lived up to now.

RECOMMENDED READING

Dean, C. *Hormone Balance.* Avon, Massachusettes: Adams Media, 2005.

Levy, T. E. *Stop America's #1 Killer: Reversible Vitamin Deficiency Found to Be Origin of ALL Coronary Heart Disease.* Henderson, NV: Livon Books, 2006.

CHAPTER 12

PROTECT YOURSELF FROM CANCER:

REDUCING YOUR RISK OF BREAST, OVARIAN, ENDOMETRIAL, AND CERVICAL CANCERS

"There is no magic bullet. There is no monotherapy that cures cancer . . . but there is a lifestyle change that prevents, arrests, and reverses serious chronic disease."
—ANDREW W. SAUL, PH.D., *FOODMATTERS*

If there is one word a doctor can say that can shake us to the core, it's *cancer.* It's real. It's scary. It changes everything.

Let's try to make that moment never happen.

According to the National Cancer Institute, over 290,000 women in the United States will be diagnosed with breast, cervical, ovarian, endometrial, vaginal, or vulvar cancer this year.[1] We will turn to the top medical doctors and brightest scientific minds. We will check into some of the most advanced medical facilities in the country. We will depend on intensive treatment options consisting predominately of chemotherapy, radiation, and surgery.

And, this year, over 67,000 women will die anyway.[2]

It's no wonder that the word cancer is synonymous with "evil." When dealing with a topic so dark, it's very hard to see the bright side. But there is one. Better nutrition can save lives—tens of thousands of them. In a recent report submitted to the President of the

United States, the National Cancer Institute stated that unhealthy diets account for a third of all cancer deaths in America.[3] Cancer is killing over half a million people in the United States each year, meaning that there are thousands upon thousands of preventable deaths. We can do something about this.

There are steps you can take *right now* that reduce your risk of getting cancer. There are changes you can make *right now* to help improve the way you feel, and keep you healthy in the long run.

TIPS TO REDUCE RISK: WHAT TO STOP DOING

Cancer should not be a game of wait-and-see. We have to choose to live our lives *now* in a way that decreases our risk of sickness in the future. We can't take away all risk, but we can make cancer a whole lot less likely. The benefits of healthy living are obvious. Better nutrition and a better lifestyle will improve the way we feel right now and, at the same time, minimize the chance that we will be in the doctor's office later. The frightening part is, if we don't invest the time today to better our health, we may be investing in cancer instead. Let's set ourselves up for success; let's live knowing that we are doing everything we can to keep cancer away.

Cut the Fat

There is a significant connection between high dietary fat intake and the risk of breast, ovarian, and endometrial cancer,[4] specifically from animal sources like red meat.[5] Colorectal cancer, which ranks second or third as the most common cancer killer of women in America depending on your race, is strongly linked with high intakes of animal fat.[6] On average, each one of us is downing about 114 pounds of red meat every year, an amount way out of proportion to our intake of fruits and vegetables.[7] What comes along with ingesting all these dead animal parts? A large amount of saturated fat. In countries like ours, where a hefty amount of calories in our diet are due to fat, the incidence of breast cancer is greater than in countries that consume much less.[8]

Reduce Your Alcohol Intake and Stop Smoking

If you drink, especially on a regular basis, you may be increasing your risk of breast and ovarian cancer.[9] And you already know about smoking. "Cancer" and "smoking" are words that have been in bed together for some time. Since smoking is potentially doubling your risk for ovarian cancer, quitting sooner rather than later is a good idea.[10] If you stop smoking, your risk for ovarian cancer returns to normal in the long term, once twenty or thirty years have gone by.[11] Smoking also increases your risk of cervical cancer,[12] and breast cancer,[13] especially if you started lighting up before you were seventeen.[14]

Ditch the Pill

Hundreds more women will get cancer each year because they are taking oral contraceptives.[15] Perhaps this seems inconsequential in comparison to the multitude of women who will take the pill and not get sick. As far as I'm concerned, a potentially lethal disease just does not need any encouragement. Taking oral contraceptives may not be worth the trade-off, especially since cancer is just one serious side effect of a drug plagued with plenty of others.

Reduce Your Intake of Sugar

Regularly eating foods that cause your blood sugar to spike, such as sugary, processed junk foods, are associated with ovarian, endometrial, and breast cancer risk.[16]

TIPS TO REDUCE RISK: WHAT TO START DOING

Health insurance is more useful for the sick: it's substantially more about paying for treatment than it's ever been about prevention. Not needing treatment is far better. What you really need is "nutritional insurance," a term coined over fifty years ago by Robert J. Williams, Ph.D., discoverer of pantothenic acid (B_5). To take out this insurance policy, you'll need to take your vitamins and adopt healthy lifestyle choices . . . right now.

Invest in Nutritional Insurance

Nutritional insurance starts with eating more fruits and vegetables. Lots more, especially those that are rich in carotenoids, lycopenes, and antioxidants. Tomatoes, green vegetables like broccoli, carrots, cabbage, yams, red, orange and yellow fruits—all are good choices. Government guidelines indicate that Americans should be getting five to nine servings or more of fruits and vegetables every day.[17] (Take it a step further, and make those *raw* fruits and veggies.) This really isn't all that much. Five servings measures out to be about two and a half cups of food or the equivalent of about one apple, twelve baby carrots, and four large strawberries.[18] Most of us don't even manage that. Only about 30 percent of us getting the recommended amount of either two servings of fruit *or* three servings of vegetables,[19] and only 11 percent of Americans are meeting U.S. Department of Agriculture (USDA) guidelines for both.[20] Surveys have found that there are a whopping 20 percent of folks out there that eat absolutely no veggies *at all*.[21] We don't even have to measure and count anymore. The USDA now recommends making half of your plate fruits and vegetables.[22] Look down and see what's there. A recommendation can't get much clearer than that. We must eat more of the right kinds of food; and when we eat more of the right stuff, we eat less of what we shouldn't. Our stomach is only so big! Eating a lot of fruits and vegetables can protect us against many cancers[23] and chronic diseases.[24] In fact, a higher intake of fruits and vegetables can cut your risk of cancer approximately in *half*.[25] That's pretty darn significant.

Sometimes what makes the most sense seems to be what folks rebel against. This is all too evident when looking at cancer patient research. The people that may be most in need of good food are probably not eating it. One study that looked at 9,105 cancer survivors and found only 15 to 19 percent were meeting the old five-a-day fruit and vegetable recommendation.[26] They are eating even worse than the rest of us.

Perhaps there is a reason for the lack of healthy choices. Perhaps fresh fruits and vegetables are just too expensive. In a report from the USDA, a consumer could buy three servings of fruit and four servings of vegetables for an amount that is less than the cost of a candy bar.[27] Their suggested fruit and veggie budget measures out to be about 12 to 16 percent of a person's daily food expenditures, leaving well over 80 percent of the grocery budget for other foods, even in low-income households.[28] If that number is even close to accurate, then it's hard to argue that cost is the issue.

Okay, what about availability? Perhaps we just don't have access to healthy food. According to a 2009 report from the USDA, 2.2 percent of American households (without access to a car) live more than one mile from a supermarket and another 3.4 percent without car access live half a mile to a mile away.[29] This means that there are millions of folks out there who may not have easy access to nutritious food. But what about the other 95 percent of American households? What's their excuse? Apparently, even when access is improved, there is little to no change in consumption of healthy foods.[30]

So, it's not really about cost, and it's not really about access. What is far more likely is that we are just set in our dietary ways. Maybe we just choose not to eat what we know to be good for us. It's time for a change.

EAT YOGURT AND GET MORE FIBER

Women who consumed probiotics, namely lactobacilli or bifidobacteria, showed an inverse relationship with the incidence of breast cancer.[31] Probiotics might offer some protection from other forms of cancer, too.[32]

In addition to the nutrients they offer, eating fruits and vegetables will help you get fiber into your diet, which is an important piece of your nutritional insurance. High-fiber diets are associated with a reduced risk of breast, ovarian, and endometrial cancers.[33]

Exercise

Oh, my gosh, we need to *move*. Staying active is so very important. Whether we are young or old, exercise is associated with a reduced risk of breast, endometrial, and ovarian cancers.[34] Keeping excess weight off will help reduce the risk of these cancers, too.[35]

Take Your Vitamins

Vitamins do not replace a good diet, but for some people, darn it, they may be all they've got. Even conscientious eaters may have difficulty consistently providing their bodies with enough of the good stuff, and that's where supplemental vitamins come in. Supplements are essential in a world where people regularly do not eat what they should, and I argue that this is true even for the folks who do.

VITAMINS THAT ARE PROTECTIVE AGAINST CANCER

Let's go one step better than a balanced diet. I'm recommending that you not only eat healthy meals but you also take your vitamins. That's a one-two punch that cancer won't be able to beat easily. Vitamins that are protective against cancer include A, C, D, E, and the Bs. Helpful minerals include selenium, zinc, and magnesium.

Vitamin A and Beta-Carotene

There is no doubt about it: folks who don't get enough vitamin A are more apt to develop cancer.[36] Specifically of note for us ladies, more vitamin A may mean a reduced risk of endometrial cancer[37] and other studies have shown significant associations between higher intakes of beta-carotene and a lower risk of breast and cervical cancers.[38]

The best way to get your "A" is through the carotene in foods like carrots, winter squash, spinach, cantaloupe, and pumpkin. Juicing fresh, raw vegetables provides you with a blast of healthy beta-carotene in quantity that's (literally) easier to swallow. Your body will absorb carotene and then make just the right amount of retinol A that your body requires at any moment. For those folks who aren't going to buy (and actually use) a juicer, supplementing with an immune-enhancing 5,000–10,000 international units (IU) of the nutrient in supplement form would be wise.

Believe it or not, there are those who will tell you that vitamin A might stimulate the growth of breast cancer.[39] Don't toss out those carrots just yet. What the study actually said was that vitamin A can cause some cells to develop blood vessels. That's a long way from promoting cancer. Just developing blood vessels doesn't mean you are causing cancer. Let it be heard loud and clear: vitamin A does not cause cancer. Indeed, it does just the opposite. "Studies in cell culture and animal models have documented the capacity for natural and synthetic retinoids to reduce carcinogenesis significantly in skin, breast, liver, colon, prostate, and other sites," states the Linus Pauling Institute.[40] The bunnies have been right all along.

Vitamin C

Along with A, you are going to want to take vitamin C, too. Vitamins work better together. Just providing your body with one nutrient is about as logical as eating only one type of food every meal, every day: it isn't. In a study involving cultured human breast cancer cells, vitamins A and C worked three times better together to prevent cancer cell proliferation than they did when administered separately.[41] Getting an average of just 110–205 milligrams (mg) of vitamin C a day is associated with a 39 to 63 percent reduced risk of breast cancer, as compared to women who get less vitamin C (31–70 mg per day).[42] I'm going to recommend that you take more than that. Much more. I agree with the two-time Nobel Prize-winning scientist Linus Pauling, who recommended 6,000–18,000 mg of vitamin C a day.[43] Your optimum dosage may be more or less, depending on your needs and comfort level. Worried about kidney stones? Don't be. The Orthomolecular Medicine News Service reports: "There is no evidence that vitamin C causes kidney stones. Indeed, in some cases, high doses may be curative. A recent, large-scale, prospective study followed 85,557 women for 14 years and found no evidence that vitamin C causes kidney stones. There was no difference in the occurrence of stones between people taking less than 250 milligrams per day and those taking 1.5 grams or more."[44]

"WAIT. I READ IN THE NEWS THAT TAKING A MULTIVITAMIN IS RISKY."

For those of you concerned that a daily multivitamin doesn't help, or even harms your health, let's put your mind at ease. With an article entitled "What Kind of Medical Study Would Have Grandma Believe that Her Daily Multivitamin Is Dangerous?" the Orthomolecular Medicine News Service (OMNS) responds to a recent study that would have us believing we should be lining up in our local grocer's returns department with our vitamin bottles.[46]

WHAT KIND OF MEDICAL STUDY WOULD HAVE GRANDMA BELIEVE THAT HER DAILY MULTIVITAMIN IS DANGEROUS?

by Robert G. Smith, Ph.D.

(OMNS, Oct 12, 2011) A newly released study suggests that multivitamin and nutrient supplements can increase the mortality rate in older women.[1] However, there are several concerns about the study's methods and significance.

- The study was observational, in which participants filled out a survey about their eating habits and their use of supplements. It reports only a small increase in overall mortality (1%) from those taking multivitamins. This is a small effect, not much larger than would be expected by chance. Generalizing from such a small effect is not scientific.

- **The study actually reported that taking supplements of B-complex, vitamins C, D, E, and calcium and magnesium were associated with a *lower* risk of mortality.** But this was not emphasized in the abstract, leading the non-specialist to think that all supplements were associated with mortality. The report did not determine the amounts of vitamin and nutrient supplements taken, nor whether they were artificial or natural. Further, most of the association with mortality came from the use of iron and copper supplements, which are known to be potentially inflammatory and toxic when taken by older people, because they tend to accumulate in the body.[2,3,4] The risk from taking iron supplements should not be generalized to imply that all vitamin and nutrient supplements are harmful.

- The study lacks scientific plausibility for several reasons. It tabulated results from surveys of 38,000 older women, based on their recall of what they ate over an 18-year period. But they were only surveyed 3 times during that period, relying only on their memory of what foods and supplements they took. This factor alone causes the study to be unreliable.

- Some of these women smoked (~15%) or had previously (~35%), some drank alcohol (~45%), some had high blood pressure (~40%), and many of them developed heart disease and/or cancer. Some preexisting medical conditions were taken into account by adjusting the risk factors, but this caused the study to contradict what we already know about efficacy of supplements. For example, the study reports an increase in mortality from taking vitamin D, when adjusted for several health-relevant factors. However, vitamin D has recently been clearly shown to be helpful in preventing heart disease[5] and many types of cancer,[6] which are major causes of death. Furthermore, supplement users were twice as likely to be on hormone replacement therapy, which is a more plausible explanation for increased mortality than taking supplements.

- The effect of doctor recommendations was not taken into account. By their own repeated admissions, **medical doctors and hospital nutritionists are more likely to recommend a daily multivitamin, and only a multivitamin, for their sicker patients**. The study did not take this into account. All it did was tabulate deaths and attempt to correct the numbers for some prior health conditions. The numbers reported do not reflect other factors such as developing disease, side effects of pharmaceutical prescriptions, or other possible causes for the mortality. The study only reports statistical correlations, and gives no plausible cause for a claimed increase in mortality from multivitamin supplements.

- The effect of education was not taken into account. When a doctor gives advice about illnesses, well-educated people will often respond by trying to be proactive. Some will take drugs prescribed by the doctor, and some will try to eat a better diet, including supplements of vitamins and nutrients. This is suggested by the study itself: the supplement users in the survey had more education than those who did not take supplements. It seems likely, therefore, the participants who got sick were more likely to have taken supplements. Because those who got sick are also more likely to die, it stands to reason that they would also be more likely to have taken supplements. This effect is purely statistical; it does not represent an increase in risk that taking supplements of vitamins and essential nutrients will cause disease or death. This type of statistical correlation is very common in observational health studies and those who are health-conscious should not be confounded by it.

- The known safety of vitamin and nutrient supplements when taken at appropriate doses was not taken into account. The participants most likely took a simple multivitamin tablet, which contains low doses. Much higher doses are also safe,[4,7] implying that the low doses in common multivitamin tablets are very safe. Further, because each individual requires different amounts of vitamins and nutrients, some people must take much higher doses for best health.[8]

Summary: In an observational study of older women in good health, it was said that those who died were more likely to have taken multivitamin and nutrient supplements than those who did not. The effect was small, and does not indicate any reason for disease or death. Instead, the study's methods suggest that people who have serious health conditions take vitamin and mineral supplements because they know that supplements can help. Indeed, the study showed a benefit from taking B-complex, C, D, and E vitamins, and calcium and magnesium. Therefore, if those wanting better health would take appropriate doses of supplements regularly, they would likely continue to achieve better health and longer life.

(Robert G. Smith is Research Associate Professor, University of Pennsylvania Department of Neuroscience. He is a member of the Institute for Neurological Sciences and the author of several dozen scientific papers and reviews.)

REFERENCES [NUMBERED AS IN ORIGINAL SOURCE]

1. Mursu, J., K. Robien, L. J. Harnack, et al. "Dietary Supplements and Mortality Rate in Older Women. The Iowa Women's Health Study." *Arch Intern Med* 171(18) (Oct 10, 2011):1625–1633.

2. Emery, T. F. *Iron and your Health: Facts and Fallacies.* Boca Raton, FL: CRC Press, 1991.

3. Fairbanks, V. F. "Iron in Medicine and Nutrition." Chapter 10 in *Modern Nutrition in Health and Disease,* editors M. E. Shils, J. A. Olson, M. Shike, et al., 9th ed. Baltimore, MD: Williams & Wilkins, 1999.

4. Hoffer, A., A. W. Saul. *Orthomolecular Medicine for Everyone: Megavitamin Therapeutics for Families and Physicians.* Laguna Beach, CA: Basic Health Publications, 2008.

5. Parker, J., O. Hashmi, D. Dutton, et al. "Levels of Vitamin D and Cardiometabolic Disorders: Systematic Review and Meta-Analysis. *Maturitas.* 65(3) (Mar 2010):225–236.

6. Lappe, J. M., D. Travers-Gustafson, K. M. Davies, et al. "Vitamin D and Calcium Supplementation Reduces Cancer Risk: Results of a Randomized Trial. *Am J Clin Nutr* (Jun 2007) 85(6):1586–1591.

7. Padayatty, S. J., A. Y. Sun, Q. Chen, et al. "Vitamin C: Intravenous Use by Complementary and Alternative Medicine Practitioners and Adverse Effects." *PLoS One* 5(7) (Jul 7, 2010):e11414.

8. Williams. R. J., G. Deason. "Individuality in Vitamin C Needs. *Proc Natl Acad Sci USA* 57(6) (Jun 1967):1638–1641.

You can find this article and more at http://orthomolecular.org/resources/omns/index.shtml, and subscribe to the Orthomolecular Medicine News Service (for free) at http://orthomolecular.org/subscribe.html.

A Good Multivitamin

Believe it: the multivitamin your mother took helped you not get childhood cancer. A review that looked at research dating back from 1960 all the way up to 2005 found "maternal ingestion of prenatal multivitamins is associated with a decreased risk for pediatric brain tumors, neuroblastoma, and leukemia."[45] Prenatal vitamins aren't just a tad helpful; they cut cancer risk in children up to 47 percent. If multivitamins help protect our unborn children from disease, it's fair to assume they do the same for us.

Vitamin D

Feel like cutting your chances of getting breast cancer in half? One study showed that generous amounts of vitamin D_3, about 2,000 IU per day, could do just that.[47] A great way to get vitamin D is through exposure to sunshine. But what do we do when we go outside? We slather on sunscreen to avoid sun damage, which is generally a good idea. But, in doing so, we block the rays that give us the vitamin we need. The solution? Be sun-block free for five to ten minutes a day a few times a week.[48]

Supplementation with vitamin D becomes especially necessary in areas of the country where so few of us get enough exposure to the sun. If you are only taking in the government-recommended daily amounts of D, it is likely that you aren't getting enough. To find out for yourself, have your doctor test the level of vitamin D in your blood at your next checkup.

Our breasts aren't the only cancer-prone area of our body that will benefit from additional vitamin D. Our ovaries will thank us, too. In areas of the country where exposure to sun is more limited, women are more prone to get ovarian cancer.[49] Previous studies have shown that not getting enough vitamin D is associated with ovarian cancer[50] and polycystic ovary syndrome.[51] A four-year trial involving 1,179 women receiving 1,400–1,500 mg of calcium and 1,100 IU of D_3 a day—that's about twice the United States Recommended Dietary Allowance (RDA)—reduced their risk of cancer by 50–60 percent, cutting their risk of all forms of cancer in half.[52]

Vitamin D really does do the body good.

Vitamin E

Vitamin E is another cancer deterrent. Getting more E is correlated with a reduction of breast and cervical cancer;[53] it may reduce your risk for endometrial cancer[54] and may substantially decrease your risk for the number-one cancer killer of women: lung cancer.[55] Lung cancer kills even more women than breast cancer.[56] Tens of thousands of these cases could be prevented if we could just gather up the strength to put the cigarettes down. If you have a girlfriend who smokes, support her in her quest to stop, and buy her a bottle of vitamin E for her birthday. (We want her to have many more of them.) One study showed that there was a massive reduction of lung cancer risk (more than half!) in people that took more vitamin E as opposed to people who took less.[57]

B Vitamins

The B vitamins are going to come in handy, too. Saul points out that "There is ever growing evidence that stress itself is a major factor in cancer—which makes sense, since stress depletes the body of B and C vitamins."[58] Sufficient amounts of B_6 and folate (B_9) may reduce your risk for colorectal cancer.[59] Folate (B_9) may also reduce your risk for endometrial cancer.[60] Evidence also shows that adequate amounts of vitamins B_{12}, B_6, and particularly folate, may help reduce your risk for breast cancer;[61] this is especially true for women who drink alcohol.[62]

Does Folic Acid Cause Cancer?

Fox News told me it does![63]

Do not be fooled by claims that folic acid, the man-made form of folate, causes cancer. This tidbit of alleged truth gained the immediate attention of the media, as does many a "vitamin causes cancer" accusation in this country, which has an information delivery system that is heavily subsidized by pharmaceutical industry advertising.

If it were true that folic acid causes cancer,[64] fortified breakfast cereals, rice, pasta, and our multivitamins are going to kill us! And, of course, Mother Nature is in on the conspiracy, too. If folate is dangerous, dark green leafy veggies must be toxic. Yep, that means our own mothers are trying to do us in with spinach, asparagus, peas, and broccoli. Children around the world, rejoice! Finally, you can tell mom that you won't eat your vegetables because they cause cancer. Of course, you'll have to give up your folic-acid fortified sugar-sweetened breakfast cereals, too.

Folic acid and folate are practically identical. Folate can be found naturally in many vegetables, fruits, and legumes, and folic acid is added to grain products because we Americans eat so darn much of them. The government figured, and rightly so, that enriching foods we actually eat with an essential vitamin means we will obtain more of it.

Folic acid helps prevent cancer, not the opposite. In a study involving over 88,000 women, those who took a multivitamin containing folic acid had a markedly lower risk of developing colon cancer than those who did not.[65] More so, folic acid is quite safe and is water-soluble,[66] so any excess simply exits your body when you urinate. You are going to have a really hard time trying to give yourself cancer with folic acid. A far easier way is just to start smoking.

Vitamins aren't cancer-causing culprits, but apparently we need to keep reminding the pubic of this fact since the media is quick to report otherwise.

MINERALS THAT ARE PROTECTIVE AGAINST CANCER

You know what vitamins you need. Let's discuss the minerals you will need too.

Calcium

Calcium shows an inverse association with breast cancer[67] and colorectal cancer.[68] That's nice, but how about this: along with 1,000 IU of vitamin D, calcium helped cut the risk for women of all forms of cancer *in half*.[69] Reduce our risk of cancer by 50 percent? That's a very good reason to make sure we get enough calcium. Calcium works with magnesium, so be sure to take both each day: 1,000–1,500 mg of calcium and 400–600 mg of magnesium.

Selenium

We don't need a whole lot of selenium, but the little we need we need a lot. Selenium is safe[70] and potentially protective against cancer.[71] Women don't need selenium as much as men do, but there is still good reason to make sure you are getting enough. For example, getting more selenium may mean getting less breast cancer,[72] and

HPV, Cervical Dysplasia, and Cancer

Human papillomavirus (HPV) is the most common sexually transmitted disease out there, because at least half, if not three-quarters of us, will get it. What a lovely thought. Fortunately for most of us, it will not cause us any trouble and go away on its own. (Phew!) However, some types of HPV can cause cancer. If you are one of the many gals with HPV who was told by your doctor that you have a cancer-causing strain, you probably panicked a little bit. Being told you *might* get cancer just isn't a settling idea.

Cervical dysplasia, a term used to describe abnormal cells that show up during a routine pap smear, is caused almost exclusively by HPV. Cervical dysplasia can be mild, moderate, or severe. The mild form may go away on its own, but moderate or severe dysplasia might need extra intervention like freezing, heating, or removal of the abnormal tissue.[78] Lower levels and lower intakes of certain nutrients like vitamins A, C, E, and folate (B$_9$) have been observed in women with cervical dysplasia,[79] suggesting an increased intake of the vitamins crucial to immune function (and therefore protective against cancer) would be helpful.

In nine out of ten cases, the body's immune system will clear up an HPV infection within two years.[80] Strengthening your body's natural defenses by adopting immunity-enhancing behaviors makes a whole lot of sense. You've heard it before: eat lots of fruits and veggies, exercise, and take your vitamins.

THE NUTRIENTS YOU NEED TO HELP FIGHT CANCER BEFORE IT STARTS

Let's strengthen our immune system so it can strengthen us. Interestingly enough, the same vitamins and minerals you use to fend off infections or fight premenstrual syndrome also happen to be protective against cancer. Well, that's fantastic! Your cancer risk-reducing supplement shopping list is going to include the same important nutrients your body needs to treat and prevent a number of feminine ailments, for less than you are probably paying for cable TV.

Vitamin A: 5,000–10,000 IU per day in the form of beta-carotene or better yet, drink fresh, raw vegetable juice made from carotene rich foods like (you guessed it) carrots!

B-complex: Take one once or twice a day that contains 25–50 mg each of B_1, B_2, B_3, and B_6, 400 micrograms of folic acid; the amounts of B_{12}, biotin, and pantothenic acid can vary.

Vitamin C: 6,000–18,000 mg per day; your optimal amount may be more or less.

Calcium: In the form of carbonate or citrate, take 1,000–1,500 mg per day.

Vitamin E: 400–800 IU per day in the form of mixed tocopherols or d-alpha tocopherol.

Vitamin D: 1,000–2,000 IU per day.

Magnesium: In the form of citrate or gluconate, take 400–600 mg per day or more as needed.

Omega-3 fatty acids: Look for a fish oil supplement that contains 900–1,000 mg total of EPA and DHA omega-3 fatty acids. Read the label! A tablet that contains 1,000 mg of fish oil may only contain 300 mg of omega-3 fatty acids. You'll want to take three of those a day to get the optimum dose.

Selenium: 55–200 micrograms a day; take with vitamin E.

Multivitamin: Don't forget a multi! Take it twice a day in addition to all the other vitamins and minerals you take. Look for one that also contains 15–30 mg of zinc.

avoiding selenium deficiency may help reduce your risk of cervical cancer.[73] For those folks with cancer, selenium may help reduce mortality rates. "Death from cancer, including lung, colorectal, and prostate cancers, is lower among people with higher blood levels or intake of selenium. In addition, the incidence of nonmelanoma skin cancer is significantly higher in areas of the United States with low soil selenium content."[74] Food sources of selenium include Brazil nuts, garlic, light turkey meat, mushrooms, liver, whole wheat, noodles, barley, eggs, and fish. Selenium supplements often come in doses of 200 micrograms (mcg), which is plenty. You can take the whole tablet each day or just break it in half to supplement a good diet with about 100 mcg. Selenium and vitamin E work very well together, so it's a good idea to take them together.[75]

Zinc

Don't forget zinc! "Although many dietary compounds have been suggested to contribute to the prevention of cancer, there is strong evidence to support the fact that zinc . . . may be of particular importance in host defense against the initiation and progression of cancer."[76] Your multivitamin should have some zinc in there. Get 15–30 mg per day.

OTHER IMPORTANT NUTRIENTS: FATTY ACIDS

Omega-3 fatty acids are another supplement you may want to put on your cancer prevention nutrient list, especially if you are not a fan of eating a lot of fish. In a study that looked at the omega-3 fatty acid intake in over 34,700 women, those women with a higher intake of omega-3 had a 26 percent reduction in breast cancer risk as compared to women who weren't getting as much.[77] That's a pretty good reason to add omega-3 to your diet.

TAKING RESPONSIBILITY FOR YOUR OWN HEALTH

If we aim to keep cancer out of our lives, we must be willing to follow through by maintaining our health. Good intentions are not enough. We have to act. We have to *do*. We have to make it happen. In the film *Foodmatters*, my dad, Andrew W. Saul, said:

> People should stop being patients and start being people. Why not be healthy and happy? Why not? You change your life, you do some exercise, you eat right you feel better. All right, that's good. You look better; that's good. You live longer; that's good. You save money; that's good . . . and you have the enormous satisfaction of having done it yourself.
>
> People think, "I don't have a medical education. I can't know this." Oh, please! How complicated is it to eat right, and drink vegetable juices, and exercise? You don't need any degree to know that. It's too simple to work: it's cheap, it's simple, it's safe, [and] it's effective. The biggest single reason why people aren't doing this is, is that it requires taking responsibility, and that is the only way out.[81]

I couldn't have said it better myself.

CANCER MANAGEMENT: FEEL BETTER AS YOU STRIVE TO GET BETTER

For women who have already been diagnosed, there are things you can do *right now* to feel better during treatment, to extend your life, and even heal. Below is a list of just a few of the natural alternative and complementary cancer treatment resources out there. Keep reading. Keep learning. Keep living.

To learn more about the natural Gerson Cancer Therapy, watch *Dying to Have Known,* a documentary that delves into the efficacy and success of this nutritional treatment. This movie is available free of charge on YouTube.com.

Alternative and Complementary Cancer Treatment Resources

Cameron, E., L. Pauling. *Cancer and Vitamin C: A Discussion of the Nature, Causes, Prevention, and Treatment of Cancer With Special Reference to the Value of Vitamin C.* Revised and Expanded Ed. Philadelphia, PA: Camino Books, 1993.

González, M. J., Miranda, J. R., Saul, A. W. *I Have Cancer: What Should I Do? Your Orthomolecular Guide for Cancer Management.* Laguna Beach, CA: Basic Health Publications, 2009.

Hoffer, A., Pauling, L. *Healing Cancer: Complementary Vitamin & Drug Treatments.* Toronto, ON: CCNM Press, 2004.

Pauling, L. *How to Live Longer and Feel Better.* Corvallis, OR: Oregon State University Press, 2006.

CHAPTER 13

BE YOUR OWN
BEST DOCTOR

"Learn and live. If you don't, you won't."
—U.S. ARMY TRAINING FILM, WORLD WAR II

Sometimes we like to be told what to do, especially when it comes to our health. It's immensely comforting when a doctor, a highly trained licensed professional, identifies our problem *and* can give us a solution. The mystifying illness no longer seems a mystery, and we have been provided with its cure. The first five minutes after a doctor's visit are the best. We feel have knowledge and hope.

Many of us will discover that our hope may be misplaced. We put our faith into pharmaceuticals, which may leave us most dissatisfied. We can choose to keep returning to the doctor, or we can choose a path leading away from the disease-medicate-disease-medicate spin cycle. This path is called *education,* and it takes bravery.

The perception that there is one drug for one disease is truly a limited view. Adding a chemical to your body does not really address the underlying cause of a condition. Similarly, there is not only one nutrient needed to cure one disease. But one of these two choices is remarkably safer, usually cheaper, and, in many cases, more effective than the other.

Why a large variety of nutrients? Because there is no such thing as monotherapy with nutrition. "One drug, one disease" is a failed legend of the drug doctor. People often ask

223

me, "What is this vitamin good for?" My answer is, "Everything." They give me "the look," but it's true nevertheless. All vitamins are important. Which wheel on your car can you do without? Which wing on an airplane can you afford to leave behind?

Why large quantities of nutrients? Because that's what does the job. You don't take the amount that you think should work; you take the amount that gets results. The first rule of building a brick wall is that you have got to have enough bricks. A sick body has exaggeratedly high needs for many vitamins. You can either meet that need, or whine about why you didn't.

But why try to cure with nutrition? Well, why not? Must a cure be medical for it to be any good? . . . I say, if one doctor's black bag is empty it does not necessarily follow that all other doctors' black bags are. Go where you can get the outcome you need. The first rule of fishing is to put your hook in the water, for that is where the fish are.

I've just given you your first semester's education in heresy. People go to health heretics not because they are stupid, but because nothing else worked, and counterculture healing often does. And, despite the huge shadow of monopolistic medicine, the cartel comprising pharmacy, government, hospitals, insurance and health education, we still live in a more or less free-market economy. Honest businesses that don't provide good return to the consumer fail, unless political influence subsidizes them (which explains the continued existence of the medical and dietetic professions). This is America, and you have the right to remain sick.

—from *Doctor Yourself: Natural Healing that Works,* by Andrew W. Saul, Ph.D.

Nobody knows you better than you. As you continue to learn about yourself and your body's unique concerns, you will constantly monitor and adjust. This is the norm rather than the exception. You will pay close attention to what is going on within yourself, and if something needs to be changed, you'll do so. The more we pay attention to our bodies, the more we read about our health, the more options we discover, the more we realize that there are many safe, natural alternatives we can take advantage of, and we don't feel so reliant on a drug-based healthcare system.

Know the illness. Know your body. Know your options for fighting back. Know that you are perfectly capable of being your own doctor. Once you know this, it may not be so scary being born female.

REFERENCES

CHAPTER 2. PMS AND OTHER PERIOD RELATED PROBLEMS

1. Stöppler, M. C., W. C. Shiel, Jr. "Premenstrual Syndrome (PMS)." MedicineNet .com, http://www.medicinenet.com/premenstrual_syndrome/article.htm. (accessed October 2011).

2. Stöppler, M. C., W. C. Shiel, Jr. "Premenstrual Dysphoric Disorder (PMDD)." MedicineNet.com, http://www.medicinenet.com/premenstrual_dysphoric_disor-der_pmdd/article.htm. (accessed October 2011).

3. Ibid.

4. Drugs.com, "Ibuprofen Side Effects." http://www.drugs.com/sfx/ibuprofen-side-effects.html. (accessed October 2011).

5. Robinson, J. C., S. Plichta, C. S. Weisman, et al. "Dysmenorrhea and Use of Oral Contraceptives in Adolescent Women Attending a Family Planning Clinic." *Am J Obstet Gynecol* 166(2) (Feb 1992):578–583. Arowojolu, A. O., M. F. Gallo, L. M. Lopez, et al. "Combined Oral Contraceptive Pills for Treatment of Acne." *Cochrane Database Syst Rev* 24(1) (Jan 24, 2007):CD004425.

6. Brown, J., P. M. O'Brien, J. Marjoribanks, et al. "Selective Serotonin Reuptake Inhibitors for Premenstrual Syndrome." *Cochrane Database Syst Rev* 2 (Apr 15, 2009):CD001396.

7. Stöppler, M. C., W. C. Shiel, Jr. "Premenstrual Dysphoric Disorder (PMDD)." MedicineNet.com, http://www.medicinenet.com/premenstrual_dysphoric_disor-der_pmdd/article.htm. (accessed October 2011).

8. Findlay, S. "Research Brief: Prescription Drugs and Mass Media Advertising." National Institute for Health Care Management Foundation (NIHCM Founda-tion), September 2000. http://www.nihcm.org/pdf/DTCbrief.pdf. (accessed Octo-ber 2011).

9. Ibid.

10. Carroll, J. "Half of Americans Currently Taking Prescription Medication."

Gallup News Service, December 9, 2005. http://www.gallup.com/poll/20365/half-americans-currently-taking-prescription-medication.aspx. (accessed October 2011).

11. Starfield, B. "Is US Health Really the Best in the World?" *JAMA* 284(4) (Jul 26, 2000):483–485.

12. Woodward, L. D. "Pharmaceutical Ads: Good or Bad for Consumers?" ABC News, February 24, 2010. http://abcnews.go.com/Business/Wellness/pharmaceutical-ads-good-bad-consumers/story?id=9925198. (accessed October 2011).

13. Brown, C. S., E. W. Freeman, F. W. Ling. "An Update on the Treatment of Premenstrual Syndrome." *Am J Managed Care* 4(2) (Feb 1998):266–278.

14. Braverman, P. K. "Premenstrual Syndrome and Premenstrual Dysphoric Disorder." *J Pediatr Adolesc Gynecol* 20(1) (Feb 2007):3–12.

15. Rossignol, A. M., H. Bonnlander. "Prevalence and Severity of the Premenstrual Syndrome. Effects of Foods and Beverages That Are Sweet or High in Sugar Content." *J Reprod Med* 36(2) (Feb 1991):131–136.

16. Dean, C. *Hormone Balance: A Woman's Guide to Restoring Health and Vitality.* Avon, MA: Adams Media, 2005.

17. Rossignol, A. M., H. Bonnlander. "Caffeine-Containing Beverages, Total Fluid Consumption, and Premenstrual Syndrome." *Am J Public Health* 80(9) (Sep 1990):1106–1110.

18. Kovacs, B. "Caffeine." MedicineNet.com, http:// www.medicinenet.com/caffeine/article.htm. (accessed October 2011).

19. Griffiths, R. R., A. L. Chausmer. "Caffeine as a Model Drug of Dependence: Recent Developments in Understanding Caffeine Withdrawal, the Caffeine Dependence Syndrome, and Caffeine Negative Reinforcement." *Nihon Shinkei Seishin Yakurigaku Zasshi* 20(5) (Nov 2000):223–231.

20. Silverman, K., S. M. Evans, E. C. Strain, et al. "Withdrawal Syndrome After the Double-Blind Cessation of Caffeine Consumption." *N Engl J Med* 327(16) (Oct 15, 1992):1109–1114.

21. Sin, C. W., J. S. Ho, J. W. Chung. "Systematic Review on the Effectiveness of Caffeine Abstinence on the Quality of Sleep." *J Clin Nurs* 18(1) (Jan 2009):13–21.

22. Hoffer, A., A. W. Saul. *The Vitamin Cure for Alcoholism.* Laguna Beach, CA: Basic Health Publications, Inc., 2009.

23. Parazzini, F., L. Tozzi, R. Mezzopane, et al. "Cigarette Smoking, Alcohol Consumption, and Risk of Primary Dysmenorrhea." *Epidemiology* 5(4) (Jul 1994): 469–472. French, L. "Dysmenorrhea in Adolescents: Diagnosis and Treatment." *Paediatr Drugs* 10(1) (2008): 1–7.

24. Chen, C., S. I. Cho, A. I. Damokosh, et al. "Prospective Study of Exposure to Environmental Tobacco Smoke and Dysmenorrhea." *Environ Health Perspect* 108(11) (Nov 2000): 1019–1022.

25. Brown, S., M. Vessey, I. Stratton. "The Influence of Method of Contraception

and Cigarette Smoking on Menstrual Patterns." *Br J Obstet Gynaecol* 95(9) (Sep 1988):905–910.

26. Bertone-Johnson, E. R., S. E. Hankinson, S. R. Johnson, et al. "Cigarette Smoking and the Development of Premenstrual Syndrome." *Am J Epidemiol* 168(8) (Oct 15, 2008):938–945.

27. Ibid.

28. Chaouloff, F. "Effects of Acute Physical Exercise on Central Serotonergic Systems." *Med Sci Sports Exerc* 29(1) (Jan 1997):58–62.

29. Lustyk, M. K., L. Widman, A. Paschane, et al. "Stress, Quality of Life and Physical Activity in Women with Varying Degrees of Premenstrual Symptomatology." *Women Health* 39(3) (2004):35–44. Daley, A. "Exercise and Premenstrual Symptomatology: A Comprehensive Review." *J Womens Health (Larchmt)* 18(6) (Jun 2009):895–899. Deuster, P. A., T. Adera, J. South-Paul. "Biological, Social, and Behavioral Factors Associated with Premenstrual Syndrome." *Arch Fam Med* 8(2) Mar-Apr 1999):122–128.

30. Masho, S. W., T. Adera, J. South-Paul. "Obesity as a Risk Factor for Premenstrual Syndrome." *J Psychosom Obstet Gynaecol* 26(1) (Mar 2005):33–39.

31. Hoffer, A., J. Prousky. *Naturopathic Nutrition: A Guide to Nutrient-Rich Food and Nutritional Supplements for Optimum Health.* Toronto, ON: CCNM Press, 2006.

32. Klenner, F. R. "Observations on the Dose and Administration of Ascorbic Acid When Employed Beyond the Range of a Vitamin in Human Pathology." *J Appl Nut* 23(3–4) (1971):61–87. Cathcart, R. F. "Vitamin C, Titrating to Bowel Tolerance, Anascorbemia, and Acute Induced Scurvy." *Med Hypotheses* 7(11) (Nov 7, 1981): 1359–1376. Hoffer, A., A. W. Saul. *Orthomolecular Medicine for Everyone: Megavitamin Therapeutics for Families and Physicians.* Laguna Beach, CA: Basic Health Publications, 2008.

33. Pauling, L. *How to Live Longer and Feel Better.* Corvallis, OR: Oregon State University Press, 2006.

34. Pauling, L. *How to Live Longer and Feel Better.* Corvallis, OR: Oregon State University Press, 2006. Hickey, S., A. W. Saul. *Vitamin C: The Real Story, the Remarkable and Controversial Healing Factor.* Laguna Beach, CA: Basic Health Publications, 2008.

35. Hoffer, A., A. W. Saul. *Orthomolecular Medicine for Everyone: Megavitamin Therapeutics for Families and Physicians.* Laguna Beach, CA: Basic Health Publications, Inc., 2008.

36. Bertone-Johnson, E. R., S. E. Hankinson, A. Bendich, et al. "Calcium and Vitamin D Intake and Risk of Incident Premenstrual Syndrome." *Arch Intern Med* 165(11) (Jun 13, 2005):1246–1252.

37. Bertone-Johnson, E. R., P. O. Chocano-Bedoya, S. E. Zagarins, et al. "Dietary Vitamin D Intake, 25-Hydroxyvitamin D_3 levels and Premenstrual Syndrome in a College-Aged Population." *J Steroid Biochem Mol Biol* 121(1–2) (2010):434–437.

38. Saul, A. W. "Interview with Michael Holick, M.D." DoctorYourself.Com, http://www.DoctorYourself.com/holick.html. (accessed October 2011).

39. Bertone-Johnson, E. R., S. E. Hankinson, A. Bendich, et al. "Calcium and Vitamin D Intake and Risk of Incident Premenstrual Syndrome." *Arch Intern Med* 165(11) (Jun 13, 2005):1246–1252.

40. Saul, A. W. "Interview with Michael Holick, M.D." DoctorYourself.Com, http://www.DoctorYourself.com/holick.html. (accessed November 2011).

41. Braverman, P. K. "Premenstrual Syndrome and Premenstrual Dysphoric Disorder." *J Pediatr Adolesc Gynecol* 20(1) (Feb 2007):3–12.

42. Barnard, N. D., A. R. Scialli, D. Hurlock, et al. "Diet and Sex-Hormone Binding Globulin, Dysmenorrhea, and Premenstrual Symptoms." *Obstet Gynecol* 95(2) (Feb 2000):245–250.

43. Dawood, M. Y. "Nonsteroidal Anti-Inflammatory Drugs and Changing Attitudes toward Dysmenorrhea." *Am J Med* 84(5A) (May 20, 1988):23–29.

44. Harel, Z. "Dysmenorrhea in Adolescents." *Ann NY Acad Sci* 1135 (Jun 2008):185–195.

45. Wong, C. L., C. Farquhar, H. Roberts, et al. "Oral Contraceptive Pill as Treatment for Primary Dysmenorrhoea." *Cochrane Database Syst Rev* 4 (2009): CD002120.

46. Wang, L., X. Wang, W. Wang, et al. "Stress and Dysmenorrhoea: A Population Based Prospective Study." *Occup Environ Med* 61(12) (Dec 2004):1021–1026.

47. Akin, M. D., K. W. Weingand, D. A. Hengehold, et al. "Continuous Low-Level Topical Heat in the Treatment of Dysmenorrhea." *Obstet Gynecol* 97(3) (Mar 2001):343–349. Akin, M., W. Price, G. Rodriguez Jr., et al. "Continuous, Low-Level, Topical Heat Wrap Therapy as Compared to Acetaminophen for Primary Dysmenorrhea." *J Reprod Med* 49(9) (Sep 2004):739–745.

48. Helms, J. M. "Acupuncture for the Management of Primary Dysmenorrhea." *Obstet Gynecol* 69(1) (Jan 1987):51–56. Witt, C. M., T. Reinhold, B. Brinkhaus, et al. "Acupuncture in Patients with Dysmenorrhea: A Randomized Study on Clinical Effectiveness and Cost-Effectiveness in Usual Care." *Am J Obstet Gynecol* 198(2) (Feb 2008):166.e1–8. Taylor, D. C. Miaskowski, J. Kohn. "A Randomized Clinical Trial of the Effectiveness of an Acupressure Device (Relief Brief) for Managing Symptoms of Dysmenorrhea." *J Altern Complement Med* 8(3) (Jun 2002): 357–370.

49. "Menstrual Cramps (Dysmenorrhea)." MedicineNet.com, http://www.medicinenet .com/menstrual_cramps/page4.htm. (accessed October 2011).

50. Lefebvre, G., O. Pinsonneault, V. Antao, et al. "Primary Dysmenorrhea Consensus Guideline." *J Obstet Gynaecol Can* 27(12) (Dec 2005):1117–1146. Davis, L. S. "Stress, Vitamin B$_6$ and Magnesium in Women with and without Dysmenorrhea: A Comparison and Intervention Study" [dissertation]. Austin, TX: University of Texas at Austin, 1988. Seifert, B., P. Wagler, S. Dartsch, et al. "[Mag-

nesium—A New Therapeutic Alternative in Primary Dysmenorrhea]." *Zentralbl Gynakol* 111(11) (1989):755–760. Fontana-Klaiber, H. and B. Hogg. "[Therapeutic Effects of Magnesium in Dysmenorrhea]." *Schweiz Rundsch Med Prax* 79(16) (Apr 17, 1990):491–494.

51. Office of Dietary Supplements. National Institutes of Health. "Magnesium." http://ods.od.nih.gov/factsheets/magnesium. (accessed October 2011).

52. Dean, C. *Hormone Balance: A Woman's Guide to Restoring Health and Vitality.* Avon, MA: Adams Media, 2005.

53. McLean, L. "Therapeutic Bath Salts and Method of Use." United States Patent.   (1999), http://www.google.com/patents?hl=en&lr=&vid=USPAT5958462&id=sfQEAAA AEBAJ&oi=fnd&dq=%22epsom+salt%22+magnesium+cramps&printsec=abstra ct#v=onepage&q&f=false. (accessed October 2011).

54. Dean, C. *Hormone Balance: A Woman's Guide to Restoring Health and Vitality.* Avon, MA: Adams Media, 2005.

55. Thys-Jacobs, S., P. Starkey, D. Bernstein, et al. "Calcium Carbonate and the Premenstrual Syndrome: Effects on Premenstrual and Menstrual Symptoms. Premenstrual Syndrome Study Group." *Am J Obstet Gynecol* 179(2) (Aug 1998): 444–452.

56. Ziaei, S. M. Zakeri, A. Kazemnejad. "A Randomised Controlled Trial of Vitamin E in the Treatment of Primary Dysmenorrhoea." *BJOG* 112(4) (Apr 2005):466–469.

57. Gokhale, L. B. "Curative Treatment of Primary (Spasmodic) Dysmenorrhoea." *Indian J Med Res* 103 (Apr 1996):227–231.

58. Werbach, M. R., J. Moss. *Textbook of Nutritional Medicine.* Tarzana, CA: Third Line Press, 1999.

59. Werbach, M. R., J. Moss. *Textbook of Nutritional Medicine.* Tarzana, CA: Third Line Press, 1999. Harel, Z., F. M. Biro, R. K. Kottenhahn, et al. "Supplementation with Omega-3 Polyunsaturated Fatty Acids in the Management of Dysmenorrhea in Adolescents." *Am J Obstet Gynecol* 174(4) (1996):1335–1338.

60. Deutch, B., E. B. Jørgensen, J. C. Hansen. "Menstrual Discomfort in Danish Women Reduced by Dietary Supplements of Omega-3 PUFA and B_{12} (Fish Oil or Seal Oil Capsules)." *Nutr Res* 20(5) (2000):621–631.

61. Davis, L. S. "Stress, Vitamin B_6 and Magnesium in Women with and without Dysmenorrhea: A Comparison and Intervention Study" [dissertation]. Austin, TX: University of Texas at Austin, 1988. Seifert, B., P. Wagler, S. Dartsch, et al. "[Magnesium—A New Therapeutic Alternative in Primary Dysmenorrhea]." *Zentralbl Gynakol* 111(11) (1989):755–760.

62. Stewart, W. F., R. B. Lipton, D. D. Celentano, et al. "Prevalence of Migraine Headache in the United States." *JAMA* 267(1) (1992):64–69.

63. Osterhaus, J. T., D. L. Gutterman, J. R. Plachetka. "Healthcare Resource and Lost Labour Costs of Migraine Headache in the US." *Pharmacoeconomics* 2(1)

(Jul 1992):67–76. Gerth, W. C., G. W. Carides, E. J. Dasbach, et al. "The Multinational Impact of Migraine Symptoms on Healthcare Utilisation and Work Loss." *Pharmacoeconomics* 19(2) (2001):197–206. Lipton, R. B., W. F. Stewart, and M. Von Korff. "Burden of Migraine: Societal Costs and Therapeutic Opportunities." *Neurology* 48(3 Suppl 3) (Mar 1997): S4–9. Von Korff, M., W. F. Stewart, D. J. Simon, et al. "Migraine and Reduced Work Performance." *Neurology* 50(6) (Jun 1998):1741–1745.

64. Facchinetti, F., G. Sances, P. Borella, et al. "Magnesium Prophylaxis of Menstrual Migraine: Effects on Intracellular Magnesium." *Headache* 31(5) (May 1991):298–301.

65. Ibid.

66. Ibid.

67. Hoffer, A., J. Prousky. *Naturopathic Nutrition: A Guide to Nutrient-Rich Food and Nutritional Supplements for Optimum Health.* Toronto, ON: CCNM Press, 2006. Schoenen, J., J. Jacquy, M. Lenaerts. "Effectiveness of High-Dose Riboflavin in Migraine Prophylaxis. A Randomized Controlled Trial." *Neurology* 50(2) (Feb 1998):466–470.

68. Werbach, M. R., J. Moss. *Textbook of Nutritional Medicine.* Tarzana, CA: Third Line Press, 1999.

69. Straumsheim, P., C. Borchgrevink, P. Mowinckel, et al. "Homeopathic Treatment of Migraine: A Double Blind, Placebo Controlled Trial of 68 Patients." *Br Homeopath J* 89(1) (Jan 2000):4–7. Ernst, E. "Homeopathic Prophylaxis of Headaches and Migraine? A Systematic Review." *J Pain Symptom Manage* 18(5) (Nov 1999):353–357.

70. Nuhn, T. R. Lüdtke, M. Geraedts. "Placebo Effect Sizes in Homeopathic Compared to Conventional Drugs - A Systematic Review of Randomised Controlled Trials." *Homeopathy* 99(1) (Jan 2010):76–82.

71. Kirby, B. J. "Safety of Homeopathic Products." *J R Soc Med* 95(5) (May 2002):221–222.

72. Looker, A. C., P. R. Dallman, M. D. Carroll, et al. "Prevalence of Iron Deficiency in the United States." *JAMA* 277(12) (1997):973–976.

73. U.S. Department of Health and Human Services. National Institutes of Health. National Heart Lung and Blood Institute. "Who Is at Risk for Iron-Deficiency Anemia?" http://www.nhlbi.nih.gov/health/health-topics/topics/ida/atrisk.html. (accessed October 2011).

74. U. S. Department of Health and Human Services. National Institutes of Health. National Heart Lung and Blood Institute. "What Are the Signs and Symptoms of Iron-Deficiency Anemia?" http://www.nhlbi.nih.gov/health/health-topics/topics/ida/signs.html. (accessed October 2011).

75. Murray-Kolb, L. E., J. L. Beard. "Iron Treatment Normalizes Cognitive Functioning in Young Women." *Am J Clin Nutr* 85(3) (Mar 2007):778–787. Bruner, A. B., A. Joffe, A. K. Duggan, et al. "Randomised Study of Cognitive Effects of

Iron Supplementation in Non-Anaemic Iron-Deficient Adolescent Girls." *Lancet* 348(9033) (Oct 12, 1996):992–996. Murray-Kolb, L. E. "Iron Status and Neuropsychological Consequences in Women of Reproductive Age: What Do We Know and Where Are We Headed?" *J Nutr* (Apr 2011) Epub.

76. Verdon, F., B. Burnand, C-L Fallab Stubi, et al. "Iron Supplementation for Unexplained Fatigue in Non-Anaemic Women: Double Blind Randomised Placebo Controlled Trial." *Brit Med J* 326(7399) (May 24, 2003):1124.

77. Cheraskin, E., W. M. Ringsdorf Jr., F. H. Medford. "Daily Vitamin C Consumption and Fatigability." *J Am Geriatr Soc* 24(3) (Mar 1976):136–137.

78. Werbach, M. R., J. Moss. *Textbook of Nutritional Medicine.* Tarzana, CA: Third Line Press, 1999. Heap, L. C., T. J. Peters, S. Wessely. "Vitamin B Status in Patients with Chronic Fatigue Syndrome." *J R Soc Med* 92(4) (Apr 1999): 183–185.

79. Cox, I. M., M. J. Campbell, D. Dowson. "Red Blood Cell Magnesium and Chronic Fatigue Syndrome." *Lancet* 337(8744) (Mar 30, 1991):757–760.

80. Werbach, M. R., J. Moss. *Textbook of Nutritional Medicine.* Tarzana, CA: Third Line Press, 1999. Werbach, M. R. "Nutritional Strategies for Treating Chronic Fatigue Syndrome." *Altern Med Rev* 5(2) (Apr 2000):93–108.

81. Dean, C. *Hormone Balance: A Woman's Guide to Restoring Health and Vitality.* Avon, MA: Adams Media, 2005.

82. Ibid.

83. Walker, A. F., M. C. Souza, M. F. Vickers, et al. "Magnesium Supplementation Alleviates Premenstrual Symptoms of Fluid Retention." *J Womens Health* 7(9) (Nov 1998):1157–1165.

84. Thys-Jacobs, S., P. Starkey, D. Bernstein, et al. "Calcium Carbonate and the Premenstrual Syndrome: Effects on Premenstrual and Menstrual Symptoms. Premenstrual Syndrome Study Group." *Am J Obstet Gynecol* 179(2) (Aug 1998): 444–452. Thys-Jacobs, S., S. Ceccarelli, A. Bierman, et al. "Calcium Supplementation in Premenstrual Syndrome: A Randomized Crossover Trial." *J Gen Intern Med* 4(3) (May-Jun 1989):183–189.

85. Yanovski, S. "Sugar and Fat: Cravings and Aversions." *J Nutr* 133(3) (Mar 2003):835S-837S. Bruinsma, K., D. L. Taren. "Chocolate: Food or Drug?" *J Am Diet Assoc* 99(10) (Oct 1999):1249–1256.

86. Office of Dietary Supplements. National Institutes of Health. "Magnesium." http://ods.od.nih.gov/factsheets/magnesium. (accessed October 2011).

87. Ibid.

88. Docherty, J. P., D. A. Sack, M. Roffman, et al. "A Double-Blind, Placebo-Controlled, Exploratory Trial of Chromium Picolinate in Atypical Depression: Effect on Carbohydrate Craving." *J Psychiatr Pract* 11(5) (Sep 2005):302–314.

89. Saul, A. W. *Doctor Yourself: Natural Healing That Works.* Laguna Beach, CA: Basic Health Publications, 2003.

90. Saul, A. W. *Doctor Yourself: Natural Healing That Works*. Laguna Beach, CA: Basic Health Publications, 2003. Anderson, R., A. Kozlovsky. "Chromium Intake, Absorption, and Excretion of Subjects Consuming Self-Selected Diets," *Am J Clin Nutr* 41(6) (Jun 1985):1177–1183. Saul, A. *Fire Your Doctor: How to be Independently Healthy*. Laguna Beach, CA: Basic Health Publications, 2005.

91. London, R. S., L. Murphy, K. E. Kitlowski, et al. "Efficacy of Alpha-Tocopherol in the Treatment of the Premenstrual Syndrome." *J Reprod Med* 32(6) (Jun 1987):400–404.

92. Thys-Jacobs, S., S. Ceccarelli, A. Bierman, et al. "Calcium Supplementation in Premenstrual Syndrome: A Randomized Crossover Trial." *J Gen Intern Med* 4(3) (May-Jun 1989):183–189.

93. Bertone-Johnson, E. R., S. E. Hankinson, A. Bendich, et al. "Calcium and Vitamin D Intake and Risk of Incident Premenstrual Syndrome." *Arch Intern Med* 165(11) (Jun 13, 2005):1246–1252.

94. Thys-Jacobs, S., S. Ceccarelli, A. Bierman, et al. "Calcium Supplementation in Premenstrual Syndrome: A Randomized Crossover Trial." *J Gen Intern Med* 4(3) (May-Jun 1989):183–189.

95. Thys-Jacobs, S., S. Ceccarelli, A. Bierman, et al. "Calcium Supplementation in Premenstrual Syndrome: A Randomized Crossover Trial." *J Gen Intern Med* 4(3) (May-Jun 1989):183–189.

96. Office of Dietary Supplements. National Institutes of Health. "Calcium." http://ods.od.nih.gov/factsheets/calcium. (accessed October 2011).

97. Thys-Jacobs, S., S. Ceccarelli, A. Bierman, et al. "Calcium Supplementation in Premenstrual Syndrome: A Randomized Crossover Trial." *J Gen Intern Med* 4(3) (May-Jun 1989):183–189. Alvir, J. M., S. Thys-Jacobs. "Premenstrual and Menstrual Symptom Clusters and Response to Calcium Treatment." *Psychopharmacol Bull* 27(2) (1991):145–148.

98. Office of Dietary Supplements. National Institutes of Health. "Calcium." http://ods.od.nih.gov/factsheets/calcium. (accessed October 2011).

99. Ibid.

100. Ibid.

101. Walker, A. F., M. C. Souza, M. F. Vickers, et al. "Magnesium Supplementation Alleviates Premenstrual Symptoms of Fluid Retention." *J Womens Health* 7(9) (Nov 1998):1157–1165.

102. London, R. S., G. S. Sundaram, L. Murphy, et al. "Evaluation and Treatment of Breast Symptoms in Patients with the Premenstrual Syndrome." *J Reprod Med* 28(8) (Aug 1983):503–508.

103. Russell, L. C. "Caffeine Restriction as Initial Treatment for Breast Pain." *Nurse Pract* 14(2) (Feb 1989):36–7, 40.

104. Werbach, M. R., J. Moss. *Textbook of Nutritional Medicine*. Tarzana, CA: Third Line Press, 1999.

105. Hoffer, A., A. W. Saul. *Orthomolecular Medicine for Everyone: Megavita-min Therapeutics for Families and Physicians.* Laguna Beach, CA: Basic Health Publications, Inc., 2008.

106. Facchinetti, F., P. Borella, G. Sances, et al. "Oral Magnesium Successfully Relieves Premenstrual Mood Changes." *Obstet Gynecol* 78(2) (Aug 1991):177–81. De Souza, M. C., A. F. Walker, P. A. Robinson, et al. "A Synergis-tic Effect of a Daily Supplement for 1 Month of 200 Mg Magnesium Plus 50 Mg Vitamin B$_6$ for the Relief of Anxiety-Related Premenstrual Symptoms: A Random-ized, Double-Blind, Crossover Study." *J Womens Health* 9(2) (Mar 2000):131–139.

107. London, R. S., L. Murphy, K. E. Kitlowski, et al. "Efficacy of Alpha-Toco-pherol in the Treatment of the Premenstrual Syndrome." *J Reprod Med* 32(6) (Jun 1987):400–404.

108. Gaby, A. R. "'Safe Upper Levels' for Nutritional Supplements: One Giant Step Backward." *J Orthomolecular Med* 18(3–4) (2003):126–130. Wyatt, K. M., P. W. Dimmock, P. W. Jones, et al. "Efficacy of Vitamin B$_6$ in the Treatment of Premenstrual Syndrome: Systemic Review." *Brit Med J* 318(7195) (May 22, 1999):1375–1381. Doll, H., S. Brown, A. Thurston, et al. "Pyridoxine (Vitamin B$_6$) and the Premenstrual Syndrome: A Randomized Crossover Trial." *J R Coll Gen Pract* 39(326) (Sep 1989):364–368.

109. Hoffer, A., J. Prousky. *Naturopathic Nutrition: A Guide to Nutrient-Rich Food and Nutritional Supplements for Optimum Health.* Toronto, ON: CCNM Press, 2006.

110. Shipowick, C. D., C. B. Moore, C. Corbett, et al. "Vitamin D and Depres-sive Symptoms in Women During the Winter: A Pilot Study." *Appl Nurs Res* 22(3) (Aug 2009):221–225.

111. Bertone-Johnson, E. R., S. E. Hankinson, A. Bendich, et al. "Calcium and Vitamin D Intake and Risk of Incident Premenstrual Syndrome." *Arch Intern Med* 165(11) (Jun 13, 2005):1246–1252. Bertone-Johnson, E. R., P. O. Chocano-Bedoya, S. E. Zagarins, et al. "Dietary Vitamin D Intake, 25-Hydroxyvitamin D$_3$ levels and Premenstrual Syndrome in a College-Aged Population." *J Steroid Biochem Mol Biol* 121(1–2) (2010):434–437.

112. Thys-Jacobs, S., S. Ceccarelli, A. Bierman, et al. "Calcium Supplementation in Premenstrual Syndrome: A Randomized Crossover Trial." *J Gen Intern Med* 4(3) (May-Jun 1989):183–189.

113. Abraham, G. E. "Nutritional Factors in the Etiology of the Premenstrual Tension Syndromes." *J Reprod Med* 28(7) (Jul 1983):446–464.

114. Ibid.

115. Gaby, A. R. "'Safe Upper Levels' for Nutritional Supplements: One Giant Step Backward." *J Orthomolecular Med* 18(3–4) (2003):126–130. Wyatt, K. M., P. W. Dimmock, P. W. Jones, et al. "Efficacy of Vitamin B$_6$ in the Treatment of Premenstrual Syndrome: Systemic Review." *Brit Med J* 318(7195) (May 22,

1999):1375–1381. Doll, H., S. Brown, A. Thurston, et al. "Pyridoxine (Vitamin B$_6$) and the Premenstrual Syndrome: A Randomized Crossover Trial." *J R Coll Gen Pract* 39(326) (Sep 1989):364–368.

116. Cohen, M., A. Bendich. "Safety of Pyridoxine—A Review of Human and Animal Studies." *Toxicol Lett* 32(2–3) (Dec 1986):129–139.

117. Gaby, A. R. "'Safe Upper Levels' for Nutritional Supplements: One Giant Step Backward." *J Orthomolecular Med* 18(3–4) (2003):126–130. Saul, A. *Fire Your Doctor: How to be Independently Healthy.* Laguna Beach, CA: Basic Health Publications, 2005. Pauling, L. *How to Live Longer and Feel Better.* Corvallis, OR: Oregon State University Press, 2006.

118. Gaby, A. R. "'Safe Upper Levels' for Nutritional Supplements: One Giant Step Backward." *J Orthomolecular Med* 18(3–4) (2003):126–130.

119. Challem, J. *The Food-Mood Solution: All-Natural Ways ato Banish Anxiety, Depression, Anger, Stress, Overeating, and Alcohol and Drug Problems—And Feel Good Again.* Hoboken, NJ: John Wiley, 2007.

120. Ohayon, M. M. "Epidemiology of Insomnia: What We Know and What We Still Need to Learn." *Sleep Med Rev* 6(2) (Apr 2002):97–111.

121. Office of Dietary Supplements. National Institutes of Health. "Magnesium." http://ods.od.nih.gov/factsheets/magnesium. (accessed October 2011).

122. Dean, C. *Hormone Balance: A Woman's Guide to Restoring Health and Vitality.* Avon, MA: Adams Media, 2005. Office of Dietary Supplements. National Institutes of Health. "Magnesium." http://ods.od.nih.gov/factsheets/magnesium. (accessed October 2011).

123. King, D. E., A. G. Mainous III, M. E. Geesey, et al. "Dietary Magnesium and C-Reactive Protein Levels." *J Am Coll Nutr* 24(3) (Jun 2005):166–171.

124. Ford, E. S., A. H. Mokdad. "Dietary Magnesium Intake in a National Sample of US Adults." *J Nutr* 133(9) (Sep 2003):2879–2882.

125. Office of Dietary Supplements. National Institutes of Health. "Magnesium." http://ods.od.nih.gov/factsheets/magnesium. (accessed October 2011).

126. Dean, C. *Hormone Balance: A Woman's Guide to Restoring Health and Vitality.* Avon, MA: Adams Media, 2005.

127. Johnson, S. "The Multifaceted and Widespread Pathology of Magnesium Deficiency." *Med Hypotheses* 56(2) (Feb 2001):163–170.

128. Ibid.

129. Prevention Health Books. *Prevention's Best Vitamin Cures: The Ultimate Compendium of Vitamin and Mineral Cures with More than 500 Remedies for Whatever Ails You!.* New York: Rodale; St. Martin's Paperbacks, 2000.

130. Prevention Health Books. *Natural Prescriptions for Women: What to Do—And When to Do It—To Solve More than 100 Female Health Problems—Without Drugs.* New York: Rodale, 1998.

131. Ibid.

132. Bronstein A.C., D.A. Spyker, L.R, Cantilena Jr, et al. "2009 Annual Report of the American Association of Poison Control Centers' National Poison Data System (NPDS): 27th Annual Report." *Clin Toxicol* 48(10) (Dec 2010):979–1178. Available at: http://www.aapcc.org/dnn/Portals/0/2009%AR.pdf. (accessed October 2011).

133. Orthomolecular Medicine News Service. "23 Years of Documented Vitamin Safety." February 27, 2007. http://orthomolecular.org/resources/omns/ v03n04 .shtml (accessed October 2011).

134. Orthomolecular Medicine News Service. "No Deaths from Vitamins—None at All in 27 Years." June 14, 2011. http://orthomolecular.org/resources/ omns/v07n05.shtml (accessed October 2011).

135. Saul, A. W., C. Gerson, D. Rogers, et al. *Foodmatters* [DVD]. Permacology Productions, 2008.

136. Saul, A. W. "The Doctor Yourself Newsletter." 4(20) September 20, 2004. http://www.DoctorYourself.com/news/v4n20.html. (accessed October 2011).

137. WebMD, "Premenstrual Syndrome (PMS) Medications." http://women .webmd.com/pms/premenstrual-syndrome-pms-medications. (accessed October 2011).

CHAPTER 3. YEAST INFECTIONS

1. Wilson, C. "Recurrent Vulvovaginitis Candidiasis; An Overview of Traditional and Alternative Therapies." *Adv Nurs Pract* 13(5) (May 2005):24–29. Marrazzo, J. "Vulvovaginal Candidiasis." *Brit Med J* 326 (May 2003): 993–994. Weissenbacher, T. M., S. S. Witkin, A. Gingelmaier, et al. "Relationship Between Recurrent Vulvovaginal Candidosis and Immune Mediators in Vaginal Fluid." *Eur J Obstet Gynecol Reprod Biol* 144(1) (May 2009):59–63.

2. RxList. The Internet Drug Index. "Monistat Vaginal Cream Side Effects." http://www.rxlist.com/monistat_vaginal_cream-drug.htm. (accessed October 2011).

3. Reid, G., and J. Burton. "Use of Lactobacillus to Prevent Infection by Pathogenic Bacteria." *Microbes Infect* 4(3) (Mar 2002):319–324.

4. Marrazzo, J. "Vulvovaginal Candidiasis." *Brit Med J* 326 (May 2003): 993–994. Nyirjesy, P. "Chronic Vulvovaginal Candidiasis." *Am Fam Physician* 63:4 (2001): 697–702.

5. Nyirjesy, P. "Chronic Vulvovaginal Candidiasis." *Am Fam Physician* 63:4 (2001): 697–702.

6. Casalmir, M. J., B. Rhee. "Pfizer/Pharmacia Merger—The Biggest Just Got Bigger." (May 2003), http://library.findlaw.com/2003/May/28/132773.html. (accessed October 2011).

7. PRNewswire. United Business Media. "U.S. Court of Appeals Affirms Pfizer's Six-Month Exclusivity for Diflucan." (April 28, 2004), http://www.prnewswire

.com/cgi-bin/stories.pl?   ACCT=104&STORY=/www/story/04–28–2004/ 0002161861&EDATE=. (accessed October 2011).

8. RxList. The Internet Drug Index. "Monistat Vaginal Cream Side Effects." http://www.rxlist.com/monistat_vaginal_cream-drug.htm. (accessed October 2011).

9. Lynch, M.E., J. D. Sobel, P. L. Fidel, Jr. "Role of Antifungal Drug Resistance in the Pathogenesis of Recurrent Vulvovaginal Candidiasis." *J Med Vet Mycol* 34(5) (1996):337–339.

10. Wilson, C. "Recurrent Vulvovaginitis Candidiasis; An Overview of Traditional and Alternative Therapies." *Adv Nurs Pract* 13(5) (May 2005):24–29. Cassone, A., F. De Barnardis, G. Santoni. "Anticandidal Immunity and Vaginitis: Novel Opportunities for Immune Intervention." *Infect Immun* 75(10) (Oct 2007):4675–4686. Richter, S. S., R. P. Galask, S. A. Messer, et al. "Antifungal Susceptibilities of Candida Species Causing Vulvovaginitis and Epidemiology of Recurrent Cases." *J Clin Microbiol* 43(5) (May 2005):2155–2162.

11. Horowitz, B.J., D. Giaquinta, S. Ito. "Evolving Pathogens in Vulvovaginal Ccandidiasis: Implications for Patient Care." *J Clin Pharmacol* 32(33) (Mar 1992):248–255.

12. Sobel, J. D., H. C. Wiesenfeld, M. Martens, et al. "Maintenance Fluconazole Therapy for Recurrent Vulvovaginal Candidiasis." *N Engl J Med* 351(9) (Aug 26, 2004):876–883.

13. Nyirjesy, P. "Chronic Vulvovaginal Candidiasis." *Am Fam Physician* 63:4 (2001): 697–702. Spinillo, A., L. Colonna, G. Piazzi, et al. "Managing Recurrent Vulvovaginal Candidiasis. Intermittent Prevention with Itraconazole." *J Reprod Med* 42(2) (Feb 1997):83–87.

14. Sobel, J. D., H. C. Wiesenfeld, M. Martens, et al. "Maintenance Fluconazole Therapy for Recurrent Vulvovaginal Candidiasis." *N Engl J Med* 351(9) (Aug 26, 2004):876–883.

15. RxList. The Internet Drug Index. "Diflucan (Fluconazole) Side Effects and Drug Interactions." (April 2007) http://www.rxlist.com/diflucan-drug.htm. (accessed October 2011).

16. Nyirjesy, P. "Chronic Vulvovaginal Candidiasis." *Am Fam Physician* 63:4 (2001): 697–702. Geiger, A. M., B. Foxman, J. D. Sobel. "Chronic Vulvovaginal Candidiasis: Characteristics of Women with Candida Albicans, C Glabrata and No Candida." *Genitourin Med* 71(5) (Oct 1995):304–307. Sihvo, S., R. Ahonen, H. Mikander, et al. "Self-Medication with Vaginal Antifungal Drugs: Physicians' Experiences and Women's Utilization Patterns." *J Fam Pract* 17(2) (2000):145–149. Ferris, D. G., C. Dekle, M. S. Litaker. "Women's Use of Over-the-Counter Antifungal Medications for Gynecologic Symptoms." *J Fam Pract* 42(6) (Jun 1996):595–600.

17. French, L., J. Horton, M. Matousek. "Abnormal Vaginal Discharge: Using Office Diagnostic Testing More Effectively." *J Fam Pract* 53(10) (Oct 2004):805–814.

18. Cassone, A., F. De Barnardis, G. Santoni. "Anticandidal Immunity and Vaginitis: Novel Opportunities for Immune Intervention." *Infect Immun* 75(10) (Oct 2007):4675–4686. Purkh, K., S. Khalsa. "Candida's Curse." *Herb Quarterly* (Summer 1996):18–23.

19. Jensen, H. K., P. A. Hansen, J. Blom. "Incidence of Candida Albicans in Women Using Oral Contraceptives." *Acta Obstet Gynecol Scand* 49(3) (Jan 1970):293–296. Pumpianski, R., S. Ganor. "Vulvovaginal Candidosis and Oral Contraceptives." *Mykosen* 17(8) (Aug 1974): 173–178. Willmott, F. E. "Genital Yeasts in Female Patients Attending a VD Clinic." *Br J Vener Dis* 51(2) (Apr 1975):119–122.

20. Spinillo, A., E. Capuzzo, S. Nicola, et al. "The Impact of Oral Contraception on Vulvovaginal Candidiasis." *Contraception* 51(5) (May 1995):293–297.

21. Fidel, P. L., J. Cutright, C. Steele. "Effects of Reproductive Hormones on Experimental Vaginal Candidiasis." *Infect Immun* 68(2) (Feb 2000):651–657. Dean, C. *Hormone Balance: A Women's Guide to Restoring Health and Vitality.* Avon, MA: Adams Media, 2005.

22. MacDonald, T. M., P. H. G. Beardon, M. M. McGilchrist, et al. "The Risks of Symptomatic Vaginal Candidiasis after Oral Antibiotic Therapy." *Q J Med* 86(7) (1993):419–424. Onifade, A. K. O.B. Olorunfemi. "Epidemiology of Vulvo-Vaginal Candidiasis in Female Patients in Ondo State Government Hospitals." *J Food Agric Environment* 3(1) (2005):118–119. Kirsch, D. R., R. Kelly and M. B. Kurtz. *The Genetics of Candida.* Boca Raton, FL: CRC Press, 1990.

23. Cassone, A., F. De Barnardis, G. Santoni. "Anticandidal Immunity and Vaginitis: Novel Opportunities for Immune Intervention." *Infect Immun* 75(10) (Oct 2007):4675–4686.

24. Horowitz, B.J., S.W. Edelstein, L. Lippman. "Sugar Chromatography Studies in Recurrent Candida Vulvovaginitis." *J Reprod Med* 29(7) (Jul 1984):441–443.

25. Onifade, A. K. O.B. Olorunfemi. "Epidemiology of Vulvo-Vaginal Candidiasis in Female Patients in Ondo State Government Hospitals." *J Food Agric Environment* 3(1) (2005):118–119. Bradshaw, C. S, A. N. Morton, S. M. Garland, et al. "Higher-Risk Behavioral Practices Associated with Bacterial Vaginosis Compared with Vaginal Candidiasis." *Obstet Gynecol* 106(1) (Jul 2005):105–114. Onderdonk, A. B., M. L. Delaney, P. L. Hinkson, et al. "Quantitative and Qualitative Effects of Douche Preparations on Vaginal Microflora." *Obstet Gynecol* 80(3 Pt 1) (Sep 1992):333–338.

26. Dean, C. *Hormone Balance: A Women's Guide to Restoring Health and Vitality.* Avon, MA: Adams Media, 2005.

27. Morton, R. S., S. Rashid. "Candidal Vaginitis: Natural History, Predisposing Factors and Prevention." *Proc R Soc Med* 70(Suppl 4) (1977):3–6. Chaitow, L. *Candida albicans: Could Yeast Be Your Problem?* Rochester, VT: Healing Arts Press, 1998.

28. Crook, W.G., C. Dean, E. Crook. *The Yeast Connection and Women's Health.* Jackson, TN: Professional Books, 2005.

29. Hilton, E., H. D. Isenberg, P. Alperstein, et al. "Ingestion of Yogurt Containing Lactobacillus Acidophilus as Prophylaxis for Candidal Vaginitis." *Ann Internal Med* 116(5) (Mar 1, 1992):353–357.

30. Cassone, A., F. De Barnardis, G. Santoni. "Anticandidal Immunity and Vaginitis: Novel Opportunities for Immune Intervention." *Infect Immun* 75(10) (Oct 2007):4675–4686.

31. Van Kessel, K., N. Assefi, J. Marrazzo, et al. "Common Complementary and Alternative Therapies for Yeast Vaginitis and Bacterial Vaginosis: A Systematic Review." *Obstet Gynecol Surv* 58(5) (May 2003):351–358.

32. Editors of Prevention Magazine. *Vitamin Cures: The Ultimate Compendium of Vitamin and Mineral Cures with More than 500 Remedies for Whatever Ails You.* New York, NY: Rodale, 2000.

33. Adetumbi, M., G. T. Javor, B. H. Lau. "Allium Sativum (Garlic) Inhibits Lipid Synthesis by Candida Albicans." *Antimicrob Agents Chemother* 30(3) (Sep 1986):499–501. Sandhu, D. K., M. K. Warraich, S. Singh. "Sensitivity of Yeasts Isolated from Cases of Vaginitis to Aqueous Extracts of Garlic." *Mykosen* 23(12) (Dec 1980):691–698.

34. Science Daily. "Men Do Not Cause Yeast Infections In Women, Study Finds." *Science Daily:* (Dec 19, 2003). http://www.sciencedaily.com/releases/2003/12/031219073022.htm. (accessed October 2011).

35. Schmid, J, M. Rotman, B. Reed, et al. Genetic Similarity of Candida Albicans Strains from Vaginitis Patients and Their Partners. *J Clin Microbiol* 31(1) (Jan 1993):39–46.

36. Sobel, J. D. "Pathogenesis and Treatment of Recurrent Vulvovaginal Candidiasis." *Clin Infect Dis* 14(Suppl 1) (Mar 1992):S148–153.

37. Alexander, M., H. Newmark, R. G. Miller. "Oral Beta-Carotene Can Increase the Number of OKT4 Cells in Human Blood." *Immunol Lett* 9(4) (1985):221–224.

38. Purkh, K., S. Khalsa. "Candida's Curse." *Herb Quarterly* (Summer 1996): 18–23.

39. Crook, W.G., C. Dean, E. Crook. *The Yeast Connection and Women's Health.* Jackson, TN: Professional Books, 2005. Sobel, J. D., W. Chaim, V. Nagappan, et al. "Treatment of Vaginitis Caused by *Candida Glabrata:* Use of Topical Boric Acid and Flucytosine." *Obstet Gynecol* 189(5) (Nov 2003):1297–1300. Van Kessel, K., N. Assefi, J. Marrazzo, et al. "Common Complementary and Alternative Therapies for Yeast Vaginitis and Bacterial Vaginosis: A Systematic Review." *Obstet Gynecol Surv* 58(5) (May 2003):351–358.

40. Berkson, D. L. *Natural Answers for Women's Health Questions.* New York, NY: Simon & Schuster, 2002. Crook, W.G., C. Dean, E. Crook. *The Yeast Connection and Women's Health.* Jackson, TN: Professional Books, 2005.

41. Hammer, K. A., C. F. Carson, T. V. Riley. "In-Vitro Activity of Essential Oils, in Particular Melaleuca Alternifolia (Tea Tree) Oil and Tea Tree Oil Products,

Against Candida Spp." *J Antimicrob Chemother* 42(5) (1998):591–595. Nenoff, P., U. F. Haustein, W. Brandt. "Antifungal Activity of the Essential Oil of Melaleuca Alternifolia (Tea Tree Oil) against Pathogenic Fungi in Vitro." *Skin Pharmacol* 9(6) (1996):388–394.

42. Crook, W.G., C. Dean, E. Crook. *The Yeast Connection and Women's Health.* Jackson, TN: Professional Books, 2005.

43. Ibid.

44. Ibid.

45. Fairfield, K. M., R. H. Fletcher. "Vitamins for Chronic Disease Prevention in Adults. Scientific Review." *JAMA* 287(23) (2002):3116–3126.

46. Pauling, L. *How to Live Longer and Feel Better.* Corvallis, OR: Oregon State University Press, 2006.

47. Hickey, S., A. W. Saul. *Vitamin C: The Real Story.* Laguna Beach, CA: Basic Health Publications, 2008.

48. Davis, A. *Let's Get Well.* New York, NY: Harcourt, Brace & World, 1965.

49. Semba, R. D. "Vitamin A, Immunity, and Infection." *Clin Infect Dis* 19(3) (Sep 1994):489–499. Werbach, M. R., J. Moss. *Textbook of Nutritional Medicine.* Tarzana, CA: Third Line Press, 1999.

50. Saul, A. W. *Doctor Yourself: Natural Healing That Works.* Laguna Beach, CA: Basic Health Publications, 2003.

51. Diplock, A. T. "Safety of Antioxidant Vitamins and Beta-Carotene." *Am J Clin Nutr* 62(6) (1995):1510S-1516S. Bendich, A. "The Safety of Beta-Carotene." *Nutr-Cancer* 11(4) (1988): 207–214.

52. Saul, A. W. *Fire Your Doctor: How to be Independently Healthy.* Laguna Beach, CA: Basic Health Publications, 2005.

53. Editors of Prevention Magazine. *Vitamin Cures: The Ultimate Compendium of Vitamin and Mineral Cures with More than 500 Remedies for Whatever Ails You.* New York, NY: Rodale, 2000. Hoffer, A., A. W. Saul. *Orthomolecular Medicine for Everyone: Megavitamin Therapeutics for Families and Physicians.* Laguna Beach, CA: Basic Health Publications, 2008.

54. Bendich, A. "Vitamin E and Immune Functions." *Basic Life Sci* 49 (1988):615–620. Meydani, S. N., M. P. Barklund, S. Liu, et al. "Vitamin E Supplementation Enhances Cell-Mediated Immunity in Healthy Elderly Subjects." *Am J Clin Nutr* 52(3) (Sep 1990):557–563.

55. Hoffer, A., J. Prousky. *Naturopathic Nutrition: A Guide to Nutrient-Rich Food and Nutritional Supplements for Optimum Health.* Toronto, ON: CCNM Press, 2006.

56. Purkh, K., S. Khalsa. "Candida's Curse." *Herb Quarterly* (Summer 1996): 18–23. Chaitow, L. *Candida albicans: Could Yeast Be Your Problem?* Rochester, VT: Healing Arts Press, 1998.

CHAPTER 4. BACTERIAL VAGINOSIS

1. Spiegel, C. A. "Bacterial Vaginosis." *Clin Microbiol Rev* 4(4) (Oct 1991):485–502. Eschenbach, D. A., P. R. Davick, B. L. Williams, et al. "Prevalence of Hydrogen Peroxide-Producing Lactobacillus Species in Normal Women and Women with Bacterial Vaginosis." *J Clin Microbiol* 27(2) (Feb 1989):251–256. Hill, G. B. "The Microbiology of Bacterial Vaginosis." *Am J Obstet Gynecol* 169(2 Pt 2) (Aug 1993):450–454.

2. Hill, G. B. "The Microbiology of Bacterial Vaginosis." *Am J Obstet Gynecol* 169(2 Pt 2) (Aug 1993):450–454. Peipert, J. F., A. B. Montagno, A. S. Cooper, et al. "Bacterial Vaginosis as a Risk Factor for Upper Genital Tract Infection." *Am J Obstet Gynecol* 177(5) (Nov 1997):1184–1187. Sweet, R. L. "Role of Bacterial Vaginosis in Pelvic Inflammatory Disease." *Clin Infect Dis* 20(Suppl 2) (1995): S271–275.

3. Taha, T. E., D. R. Hoover, G. A. Dallabetta, et al. "Bacterial Vaginosis and Disturbances of Vaginal Flora: Association with Increased Acquisition of HIV." *AIDS* 12(13) (Sep 10, 1998):1699–1706. Wiesenfeld, H. C., S. L. Hillier, M. A. Krohn, et al. "Bacterial Vaginosis Is a Strong Predictor of *Neisseria Gonorrhoeae* and *Chlamydia Trachomatis* Infection." *Clin Infect Dis* 36(5) (2003):663–668.

4. Leitich, H., B. Bodner-Adler, M. Brunbauer, et al. "Bacterial Vaginosis as a Risk Factor for Preterm Delivery: A Meta-Analysis." *Am J Obstet Gynecol* 189(1) (Jul 2003):139–147.

5. Klebanoff, M. A., J. R. Schwebke, J. Zhang, et al. "Vulvovaginal Symptoms in Women with Bacterial Vaginosis." *Obstet Gynecol* 104(2) (Aug 2004):267–272.

6. Centers for Disease Control and Prevention (CDC). "Sexually Transmitted Diseases (STDs). Bacterial Vaginosis—CDC Fact Sheet." http://www.cdc.gov/STD/BV/ STDFact-Bacterial-Vaginosis.htm. (accessed October 2011).

7. Livengood, C. H., D. E. Soper, K. Sheehan, et al. "Comparison of Once-Daily and Twice-Daily Dosing of 0.75% Metronidazole Gel in the Treatment of Bacterial Vaginosis." *Sex Transm Dis* 26(3) (Mar 1999):137–142. Schmitt, C. J. D. Sobel, C. Meriwether. "Bacterial Vaginosis: Treatment with Clindamycin Cream Versus Oral Metronidazole." *Obstet Gynecol* 79(6) (Jun 1992):1020–1023.

8. Sobel, J. D., D. Ferris, J. Schwebke, et al. "Suppressive Antibacterial Therapy with 0.75% Metronidazole Vaginal Gel to Prevent Recurrent Bacterial Vaginosis." *Am J Obstet Gynecol* 194(5) (2006):1283–1289.

9. MacDonald, T. M., P. H. G. Beardon, M. M. McGilchrist, et al. "The Risks of Symptomatic Vaginal Candidiasis after Oral Antibiotic Therapy." *Q J Med* 86(7) (1993):419–424. Onifade, A. K. O.B. Olorunfemi. "Epidemiology of Vulvo-Vaginal Candidiasis in Female Patients in Ondo State Government Hospitals." *J Food Agric Environment* 3(1) (2005):118–119. Kirsch, D. R., R. Kelly and M. B. Kurtz. *The Genetics of Candida*. Boca Raton, FL: CRC Press, 1990.

10. Bradshaw, C. S., A. N. Morton, J. Hocking, et al. "High RecurrenceRates of Bacterial Vaginosis over the Course of 12 Months after Oral Metronidazole Ther-

apy and Factors Associated with Recurrence." *J Infect Dis* 193(11) (Jun 1, 2006):1478–1486.

11. McLean, N. W., I. J. Rosenstein. "Characterisation and Selection of a *Lactobacillus* Species to Re-colonise the Vagina of Women with Recurrent Bacterial Vaginosis." *J Med Microbiol* 49(6) (2000):543–552.

12. Bradshaw, C. S., A. N. Morton, J. Hocking, et al. "High Recurrence Rates of Bacterial Vaginosis over the Course of 12 Months after Oral Metronidazole Therapy and Factors Associated with Recurrence." *J Infect Dis* 193:11 (2006):1478–1486. Baylson, F. A., P. Nyirjesy, M. V. Weitz. "Treatment of Recurrent Bacterial Vaginosis with Tinidazole." *Obstet Gynecol* 104(5 Pt 1)(Nov 2004):931–932. Hay, P. "Recurrent Bacterial Vaginosis." *Curr Infect Dis Rep* 2(6) (Dec 2000):506–512.

13. Ostrzenski, A. Gynecology: *Integrating Conventional, Complementary, and Natural Alternative Therapy*. Philadelphia, PA: Lippincott Williams & Wilkins, 2002. Wewalka, G. A. Stary, B. Bosse, et al. "Efficacy of Povidone-Iodine Vaginal Suppositories in the Treatment of Bacterial Vaginosis." *Dermatology* 204(Suppl 1) (2002):79–85. Papanikolaou, E. G., G. Tsanadis, N. Dalkalitsis, et al. "Recurrent Bacterial Vaginosis in a Virgin Adolescent: A New Method of Treatment." *Infection* 30(6) (Dec 2002):403–404. Petersen, E. E., E. R. Weissenbacher, P. Hengst, et al. "Local Treatment of Vaginal Infections of Varying Etiology with Dequalinium Chloride or Povidone Iodine. A Randomised, Double-Blind, Active-Controlled, Multicentric Clinical Study." *Arzneimittelforschung* 52(9) (2002):706–715.

14. MedicineNet.com Drug facts for metronidazole and clindamycin from www.medicinenet.com. (accessed October 2011).

15. Ibid.

16. Stöppler, M. C., W. C. Shiel, Jr. "Bacterial Vaginosis." MedicineNet.com. http://www .medicinenet.com/bacterial_vaginosis/article.htm. (accessed October 2011).

17. MedicineNet.com. Drug facts for metronidazole and clindamycin from http://www .medicinenet.com. (accessed October 2011).

18. Ness, R. B., S. L. Hillier, H. E. Richter, et al. "Douching in Relation to Bacterial Vaginosis, Lactobacilli, and Facultative Bacteria in the Vagina." 100(4) *Obstet Gynecol* (Oct 2002):765.

19. Alnaif, B., H. P. Drutz. "The Association of Smoking with Vaginal Flora, Urinary Tract Infection, Pelvic Floor Prolapse, and Post-Void Residual Volumes."*J Low Genit Tract Dis* 5(1) (Jan 2001):7–11.

20. U. S. Department of Health and Human Services Office on Women's Health. "Bacterial Vaginosis Fact Sheet." http://www.womenshealth.gov/publications/our-publications/fact-sheet/bacterial-vaginosis.cfm. (accessed October 2011).

21. Centers for Disease Control and Prevention (CDC). "Sexually Transmitted

Diseases (STDs). Bacterial Vaginosis—CDC Fact Sheet." http://www.cdc.gov/STD/BV/STDFact-Bacterial-Vaginosis.htm. (accessed October 2011).

22. Hamrick, M., M. L. Chambliss. "Bacterial Vaginosis and Treatment of Sexual Partners." *Arch Fam Med* 9(7) (Jul 2000):647–648. Vutyavanich, T., P. Pongsuthirak, P. Vannareumol, et al. "A Randomized Double-Blind Trial of Tinidazole Treatment of the Sexual Partners of Females with Bacterial Vaginosis." *Obstet Gynecol* 82(4 Pt 1) (Oct 1993):550–554.

23. Bradshaw, C. S., A. N. Morton, J. Hocking, et al. "High RecurrenceRates of Bacterial Vaginosis over the Course of 12 Months after Oral Metronidazole Therapy and Factors Associated with Recurrence." *J Infect Dis* 193(11) (Jun 1, 2006):1478–1486. Hay, P. "Recurrent Bacterial Vaginosis." *Curr Infect Dis Rep* 2(6) (Dec 2000):506–512. U. S. Department of Health and Human Services Office on Women's Health. "Bacterial Vaginosis Fact Sheet." http://www.womenshealth.gov/publications/our-publications/fact-sheet/bacterial-vaginosis.cfm. (accessed October 2011).

24. Dean, C. *Hormone Balance: A Women's Guide to Restoring Health and Vitality.* Avon, MA: Adams Media, 2005.

25. Sieber, R., and U. T. Dietz. "*Lactobacillus Acidophilus* and Yogurt in the Prevention and Therapy of Bacterial Vaginosis." *Int Dairy J* 8(7) (1998):599–607.

26. Van Kessel, K., N. Assefi, J. Marrazzo, et al. "Common Complementary and Alternative Therapies for Yeast Vaginitis and Bacterial Vaginosis: A Systematic Review." *Obstet Gynecol Surv* 58(5) (May 2003):351–358. Reid, G., A. W. Bruce, N. Fraser, et al. "Oral Probiotics Can Resolve Urogenital Infections." *FEMS Immunol Med Microbiol* 30(1) (Feb 2001):49–52. Falagas, M. E., G. I. Betsi, and S. Athanasiou. "Probiotics for the Treatment of Women with Bacterial Vaginosis." *Clin Microbiol Infect* 13(7) (Jul 2007):657–664. Saunders, S., A. Bocking, J. Challis, et al. "Effect of Lactobacillus Challenge on Gardnerella Vaginalis Biofilms." *Colloids Surf B Biointerfaces* 55(2) (Apr 1, 2007):138–142. Shalev, E., S. Battino, E. Weiner, et al. "Ingestion of Yogurt Containing Lactobacillus Acidophilus Compared with Pasteurized Yogurt as Prophylaxis for Recurrent Candidal Vaginitis and Bacterial Vaginosis." *Arch Fam Med* 5(10) (Nov-Dec 1996):593–596. Neri, A. G. Sabah, Z. Samra. "Bacterial Vaginosis in Pregnancy Treated with Yoghurt." *Acta Obstet Gynecol Scand* 72(1) (Jan 1993):17–19. Reid, G., D. Charbonneau, J. Erb, et al. "Oral Use of Lactobacillus Rhamnosus GR-1 and L. Fermentum RC-14 Significantly Alters Vaginal Flora: Randomized, Placebo-Controlled Trial in 64 Healthy Women." *FEMS Immunol Med Microbiol* 35(2) (Mar 2003):131–134. Anukam, K. C., E. Osazuwa, G. I. Osemene, et al. "Clinical Study Comparing Probiotic Lactobacillus GR-1 and RC-14 with Metronidazole Vaginal Gel to Treat Symptomatic Bacterial Vaginosis." *Microbes Infect* 8(12–13) (Oct 2006):2772–2776.

27. Anukam, K. C., E. Osazuwa, G. I. Osemene, et al. "Clinical Study Comparing Probiotic Lactobacillus GR-1 and RC-14 with Metronidazole Vaginal Gel to Treat Symptomatic Bacterial Vaginosis." *Microbes Infect* 8(12–13) (Oct 2006): 2772–2776.

28. Van Kessel, K., N. Assefi, J. Marrazzo, et al. "Common Complementary and Alternative Therapies for Yeast Vaginitis and Bacterial Vaginosis: A Systematic Review." *Obstet Gynecol Surv* 58(5) (May 2003):351–358. Reid, G., A. W. Bruce, N. Fraser, et al. "Oral Probiotics Can Resolve Urogenital Infections." *FEMS Immunol Med Microbiol* 30(1) (Feb 2001):49–52.

29. Wolf, B. W., K. B. Wheeler, D. G. Ataya, et al. "Safety and Tolerance of *Lactobacillus Reuteri* Supplementation to a Population Infected with the Human Immunodeficiency Virus." *Food Chem Toxicol* 36(12) (Dec 1998):1085–1094.

30. Anuradha, S., K. Rajeshwari. "Probiotics in Health and Disease." *J Ind Acad Clin Med* 6(1) (2005):67–72.

31. Falagas, M. E., G. I. Betsi, and S. Athanasiou. "Probiotics for the Treatment of Women with Bacterial Vaginosis." *Clin Microbiol Infect* 13(7) (Jul 2007): 657–664. Anukam, K. C., E. Osazuwa, G. I. Osemene, et al. "Clinical Study Comparing Probiotic Lactobacillus GR-1 and RC-14 with Metronidazole Vaginal Gel to Treat Symptomatic Bacterial Vaginosis." *Microbes Infect* 8(12–13) (Oct 2006):2772–2776.

32. Sobel, J. D., W. Chaim. "Treatment of Torulopsis glabrata Vaginitis: Retrospective Review of Boric Acid Therapy." *Clin Infect Dis* 24(4) (1997):649–652.

33. Ostrzenski, A. Gynecology: Integrating Conventional, Complementary, and Natural Alternative Therapy. Philadelphia, PA: Lippincott Williams & Wilkins, 2002. Van Kessel, K., N. Assefi, J. Marrazzo, et al. "Common Complementary and Alternative Therapies for Yeast Vaginitis and Bacterial Vaginosis: A Systematic Review." *Obstet Gynecol Surv* 58(5) (May 2003):351–358.

34. Ankri, S. D. Mirelman. "Antimicrobial Properties of Allicin from Garlic." *Microbes Infect* 1(2) (Feb 1999):125–129.

35. Blackwell, A. L. "Tea Tree Oil and Anaerobic (Bacterial) Vaginosis." *Lancet* 337(8736) (Feb 2, 1991):300.

36. Hammer, K. A., C. F. Carson, T. V. Riley. "In Vitro Susceptibilities of Lactobacilli and Organisms Associated with Bacterial Vaginosis to *Melaleuca Alternifolia* (Tea Tree) Oil." *Antimicrob Agents Chemother* 43(1) (Jan 1999):196.

37. Leitich, H., B. Bodner-Adler, M. Brunbauer, et al. "Bacterial Vaginosis as a Risk Factor for Preterm Delivery: A Meta-Analysis." *Am J Obstet Gynecol* 189(1) (Jul 2003):139–147.

38. Hauth, J. C., R. L. Goldenberg, W. W. Andrews, et al. "Reduced Incidence of Preterm Delivery with Metronidazole and Erythromycin in Women with Bacterial Vaginosis." *N Engl J Med* 333:26 (1995): 1732–1736. Ugwumadu, A., I. Manyonda, F. Reid, et al. "Effect of Early Oral Clindamycin on Late Miscarriage and Preterm Delivery in Asymptomatic Women with Abnormal Vaginal Flora and Bacterial Vaginosis: A Randomised Controlled Trial." *Lancet* 361(9362) (Mar 22, 2003):983–988.

39. Joesoef, M. R., S. L. Hillier, G. Wiknjosastro, et al. "Intravaginal Clindamycin Treatment for Bacterial Vaginosis: Effects on Preterm Delivery and Low Birth

Weight." *Am J Obstet Gynecol* 173(5) (Nov 1995):1527–1531. Carey, J. C., M. A. Klebanoff, J. C. Hauth, et al. "Metronidazole to Prevent Preterm Delivery in Pregnant Women with Asymptomatic Bacterial Vaginosis." *N Engl J Med* 342(8) (Feb 24, 2000):534–540. Kekki, M., T. Kurki, J. Pelkonen, et al."Vaginal Clindamycin in Preventing Preterm Birth and Peripartal Infections in Asymptomatic Women with Bacterial Vaginosis: A Randomized, Controlled Trial." *Obstet Gynecol* 97(5 Pt 1) (May 2001):643–648.

40. Reid, G., A. Bocking. "The Potential for Probiotics to Prevent Bacterial Vaginosis and Preterm Labor." *Am J Obstet Gynecol* 189(4) (Oct 2003):1202–1208.

41. Neri, A. G. Sabah, Z. Samra. "Bacterial Vaginosis in Pregnancy Treated with Yoghurt." *Acta Obstet Gynecol Scand* 72(1) (Jan 1993):17–19.

42. Hoh, J. K., H. J. Cho, S. R. Chung, et al. "The Effect of Vitamin-C Vaginal Tablets (Vagi-C(R)) in Patients with Each Vaginitis in Pregnancy and in Normal Pregnant Women." *Korean J Perinatol* 17(1) (Mar 2006):62–67.

43. Bodnar, L. M., M. A. Krohn, H. N. Simhan. "Maternal Vitamin D Deficiency is Associated with Bacterial Vaginosis in the First Trimester of Pregnancy." *J Nutr* 139(6) (Jun 2009):1157–1161.

44. Verstraelen, H., J. Delanghe, K. Roelens, et al. "Subclinical Iron Deficiency is a Strong Predictor of Bacterial Vaginosis in Early Pregnancy." *BMC Infect Dis* 5(Jul 6, 2005):55.

45. Culhane, J. F., V. Rauh, K. F. McCollum, et al. "Maternal Stress is Associated with Bacterial Vaginosis in Human Pregnancy." *Matern Child Health J* 5(2) (Jun 2001):127–134.

46. Fairfield, K. M., R. H. Fletcher. "Vitamins for Chronic Disease Prevention in Adults. Scientific Review." *JAMA* 287(23) (2002):3116–3126.

47. Semba, R. D. "Vitamin A, Immunity, and Infection." *Clin Infect Dis* 19(3) (Sep 1994):489–499.

48. Neggers, Y. H., T. R Nansel, W. W. Andrews, et al. "Dietary Intake of Selected Nutrients Affects Bacterial Vaginosis in Women." *J Nutr* 137(9) (Sep 2007):2128–2133.

49. Diplock, A. T. "Safety of Antioxidant Vitamins and Beta-Carotene." *Am J Clin Nutr* 62(6) (1995):1510S-1516S. Bendich, A. "The Safety of Beta-Carotene." *Nutr-Cancer* 11(4) (1988): 207–214.

50. Balch, J. F., P. A. Balch. *Prescription for Nutritional Healing.* New York, NY: Avery Pub. Group, 1990.

51. Ibid.

52. Hoffer, A., J. Prousky. *Naturopathic Nutrition: A Guide to Nutrient-Rich Food and Nutritional Supplements for Optimum Health.* Toronto, ON: CCNM Press, 2006.

53. Challem, J. *The Food-Mood Solution: All-Natural Ways to Banish Anxiety,*

Depression, Anger, Stress, Overeating, and Alcohol and Drug Problems—And Feel Good Again. Hoboken, NJ: John Wiley & Sons, 2007.

54. Neggers, Y. H., T. R Nansel, W. W. Andrews, et al. "Dietary Intake of Selected Nutrients Affects Bacterial Vaginosis in Women." *J Nutr* 137(9) (Sep 2007):2128–2133.

55. Fletcher, R. H., K. M. Fairfield. "Vitamins for Chronic Disease Prevention in Adults: Clinical Applications." *JAMA* 287(23) (Jun 2002):3127–3129.

56. Ibid.

57. Hillman, R. S., S. E. Steinberg. "The Effects of Alcohol on Folate Metabolism." *Annu Rev Med* 33 (1982):345–354.

58. Kaufman, W. "What Took the FDA So Long to Come Out in Favor of Folic Acid?" http://www.DoctorYourself.com/kaufman4.html. (accessed October 2011).

59. Gao X., P. E. Wilde, A. H. Lichtenstein, et al. "The Maximal Amount of Dietary Alpha-Tocopherol Intake in U.S. Adults (NHANES 2001–2002)." *J Nutr* 136(4) (2006):1021–1026. Interagency Board for Nutrition Monitoring and Related Research. *Third Report on Nutrition Monitoring in the United States.* Washington, DC: U.S. Government Printing Office, 1995.

60. Institute of Medicine. Food and Nutrition Board. *Dietary Reference Intakes: Vitamin C, Vitamin E, Selenium, and Carotenoids.* Washington, DC: National Academies Press, 2000.

61. Balch, J. F., P. A. Balch. *Prescription for Nutritional Healing.* New York, NY: Avery Pub. Group, 1990.

62. Hickey, S., A. W. Saul. *Vitamin C: The Real Story.* Laguna Beach, CA: Basic Health Publications, 2008.

63. Petersen, E. E., P. Magnani. "Efficacy and Safety of Vitamin C Vaginal Tablets in the Treatment of Non-Specific Vaginitis. A Randomised, Double Blind, Placebo-Controlled Study." *Eur J Obstet Gynecol Reprod Biol* 117(1) (Nov 2004):70–75.

64. Petersen, E. E., M. Genet, M. Caserini, et al. "Efficacy of Vitamin C Vaginal Tablets in the Treatment of Bacterial Vaginosis: A Randomised, Double Blind, Placebo Controlled Clinical Trial." *Arzneimittelforschung* 61(4) (2011):260–265.

65. Barclay, L. "Vitamin D Deficiency Linked to Bacterial Vaginosis." Medscape Medical News. Medscape Today News. http://www.medscape.com/viewarticle/703577. (accessed October 2011)

66. Office of Dietary Supplements. National Institutes of Health. "Vitamin D." http://ods.od.nih.gov/factsheets/vitamind. (accessed October 2011).

67. Ibid.

68. Neggers, Y. H., T. R Nansel, W. W. Andrews, et al. "Dietary Intake of Selected Nutrients Affects Bacterial Vaginosis in Women." *J Nutr* 137(9) (Sep 2007): 2128–2133.

69. Balch, J. F., P. A. Balch. *Prescription for Nutritional Healing.* New York, NY: Avery Pub. Group, 1990.

70. Office of Dietary Supplements. National Institutes of Health. "Magnesium." http://ods.od.nih.gov/factsheets/magnesium. (accessed October 2011).

71. Balch, J. F., P. A. Balch. *Prescription for Nutritional Healing.* New York, NY: Avery Pub. Group, 1990.

72. Solomons, N. W. "Mild Human Zinc Deficiency Produces an Imbalance Between Cell-Mediated and Humoral Immunity." *Nutr Rev* 56(1 Pt 1) (1998): 27–28. Prasad, A. S. "Zinc: An Overview." *Nutrition* 11(1 Suppl) (1995):93–99.

73. U.S. Department of Agriculture, Agricultural Research Service. "USDA Nutrient Database for Standard Reference." Release 24. http://www.nal.usda.gov/fnic/foodcomp/search/. (accessed October 2011).

74. Institute of Medicine, Food and Nutrition Board. *Dietary Reference Intakes for Vitamin A, Vitamin K, Arsenic, Boron, Chromium, Copper, Iodine, Iron, Manganese, Molybdenum, Nickel, Silicon, Vanadium, and Zinc.* Washington, DC: National Academies Press, 2001.

75. Casagrande, S. S., Y. Wang, C. Anderson, et al. "Have Americans Increased Their Fruit and Vegetable Intake? The Trends between 1988 and 2002." *Am J Prev Med* 32(4) (Apr 2007):257–263. Available online: http://www.fruitsandveggiesmorematters.org/wp-content/uploads/UserFiles/File/pdf/press/AJPM _32-4_Casagrande_with%20embargo.pdf. (accessed November 2011). Centers for Disease Control and Prevention. CDC Online Newsroom. "Majority of Americans Not Meeting Recommendations for Fruit and Vegetable Consumption." Press Release, September 29, 2009. http://www.cdc.gov/media/pressrel/2009/r090929.htm. (accessed November 2011).

CHAPTER 5. STRESS, ANXIETY, AND DEPRESSION, OH MY!

1. The National Women's Health Information Center. U. S. Department of Health and Human Services Office on Women's Health. womenshealth.gov. "Stress and Your Health Fact Sheet." http://www.womenshealth.gov/faq/stress-your-health .cfm. (accessed October 2011). Mayo Clinic Staff. "Stress Symptoms: Effects on Your Body, Feelings and Behavior." Mayo Clinic. http://www.mayoclinic.com/health/stress-symptoms/SR00008_D. (accessed October 2011).

2. Tolin, D. F., E. B. Foa. "Sex Differences in Trauma and Posttraumatic Stress Disorder: A Quantitative Review of 25 Years of Research." *Psychol Bull* 132(6) (Nov 2006):959–992.

3. The National Women's Health Information Center. U. S. Department of Health and Human Services Office on Women's Health. womenshealth.gov. "Stress and Your Health Fact Sheet." http://www.womenshealth.gov/faq/stress-your-health.cfm. (accessed October 2011).

4. Ibid.

5. Mayo Clinic Staff. "Anxiety: Risk Factors." Mayo Clinic. http://www.mayo

clinic.com/ health/anxiety/DS01187/DSECTION=risk-factors. (accessed October 2011).

6. Mayo Clinic Staff. "Anxiety: Symptoms." Mayo Clinic. http://www.mayo clinic.com/ health/anxiety/DS01187/DSECTION=symptoms. (accessed October 2011).

7. Weissman, M. M., M. Olfson. "Depression in Women: Implications for Health Care Research." *Science* 269(5225) (Aug 11, 1995):799–801.

8. Bromberger, J. T. "A Psychosocial Understanding of Depression in Women: For the Primary Care Physician." *J Am Med Womens Assoc* 59(3) (2004 Summer):198–206. Noble, R. E. "Depression in Women." *Metabolism* 54(5 Suppl 1) (May 2005):49–52.

9. Balch, J. F., P. A. Balch. *Prescriptions for Natural Healing.* New York, NY: Avery Publishing Group, 1990.

10. Mayo ClinicStaff. "Depression (Major Depression): Symptoms." Mayo Clinic. http://www.mayoclinic.com/health/depression/DS00175/DSECTION=symptoms. (accessed October 2011).

11. Chaouloff, F. "Effects of Acute Physical Exercise on Central Serotonergic Systems." *Med Sci Sports Exerc* 29(1) (Jan 1997):58–62.

12. Werbach, M. R., J. Moss. *Textbook of Nutritional Medicine.* Tarzana, CA: Third Line Press, 1999.

13. Taubes, G. "Is This Any Way to Lose Weight?" Interview. *Reader's Digest* (Feb 2011):110–119.

14. Ibid.

15. Department of Agriculture. Office of Communications. "USDA and HHS Announce New Dietary Guidelines to Help Americans Make Healthier Food Choices and Confront Obesity Epidemic." Jan 31, 2011. http://www.cnpp.usda .gov/Publications/DietaryGuidelines/2010/PolicyDoc/PressRelease.pdf. (accessed October 2011).

16. Schlebusch, L., B. A. Bosch, G. Polglase, et al. "A Double-Blind, Placebo-Controlled, Double-Centre Study of the Effects of an Oral Multivitamin-Mineral Combination on Stress." *S Afr Med J.* 90 (12) (Dec 2000):1216–1223.

17. Balch, J. F., P. A. Balch. *Prescriptions for Natural Healing.* New York, NY: Avery Publishing Group, 1990.

18. Dean, C. *Hormone Balance.* Avon, Massachusettes: Adams Media, 2005.

19. Hoffer, A., A. W. Saul. *Orthomolecular Medicine for Everyone: Megavitamin Therapeutics for Families and Physicians.* Laguna Beach, CA: Basic Health Publications, 2008. Klenner, F. R. "Observations on the Dose and Administration of Ascorbic Acid When Employed Beyond the Range of a Vitamin in Human Pathology." *J Appl Nutr* 23(3–4) (Winter 1971):61–87. Cathcart, R. F. "Vitamin C, Titrating to Bowel Tolerance, Anascorbemia, and Acute Induced Scurvy." *Med Hypotheses* 7(11) (Nov 7, 1981): 1359–1376.

20. Hoffer, A., J. Prousky. *Naturopathic Nutrition: A Guide to Nutrient-Rich Food and Nutritional Supplements for Optimum Health.* Toronto, ON: CCNM Press, 2006.

21. Pauling, L. *How to Live Longer and Feel Better.* Corvallis, OR: Oregon State University Press, 2006. Hickey, S., A. W. Saul. *Vitamin C: The Real Story.* Laguna Beach, CA: Basic Health Publications, 2008.

22. Pauling, L. *How to Live Longer and Feel Better.* Corvallis, OR: Oregon State University Press, 2006.

23. Ibid.

24. Alpert, J. E., D. Mischoulon, A. A. Nierenberg, et al. "Nutrition and Depression: Focus on Folate." *Nutrition* 16(7–8) (Jul-Aug 2000):544–546. Morris, M. S., M. Fava, P. F. Jacques, et al. "Depression and Folate Status in the US Population." *Psychother Psychosom* 72(2) (Mar-Apr 2003):80–87.

25. Abou-Saleh, M. T., A. Coppen. "The Biology of Folate in Depression: Implications for Nutritional Hypotheses of the Psychoses." *J Psychiatr Res* 20(2) (1986):91–101.

26. Wyatt, K. M., P. W. Dimmock, P. W. Jones, et al. "Efficacy of Vitamin B6 in the Treatment of Premenstrual Syndrome: Systemic Review." *Brit Med J* 318(7195) (May 22, 1999):1375–1381.

27. Challem, J. *The Food Mood Solution.* Hoboken, NJ: John Wiley & Sons, 2007.

28. Shipowick, C. D., C. B. Moore, C. Corbett, et al. "Vitamin D and Depressive Symptoms in Women During the Winter: A Pilot Study." *Appl Nurs Res* 22(3) (Aug 2009):221–225.

29. Challem, J. *The Food Mood Solution.* Hoboken, NJ: John Wiley & Sons, 2007.

30. Osher, Y, R. H. Belmaker. "Omega-3 Fatty Acids in Depression: A Review of Three Studies." *CNS Neurosci Ther* 15(2) (Jun 2009):128–133. Lin, P. Y., K. P. Su. "A Meta-Analytic Review of Double-Blind, Placebo-Controlled Trials of Antidepressant Efficacy of Omega-3 Fatty Acids." *J Clin Psychiatry* 68(7) (Jul 2007):1056–1061.

31. Szewczyk, B., E. Poleszak, M. Sowa-Ku?ma, et al. "Antidepressant Activity of Zinc and Magnesium in View of the Current Hypotheses of Antidepressant Action." *Pharmacol Rep* 60(5) (Sep-Oct 2008):588–589.

32. Rayman, M. P. "The Importance of Selenium to Human Health." *Lancet* 356(9225) (Jul 15, 2000):233–241.

33. Werbach, M. R., J. Moss. *Textbook of Nutritional Medicine.* Tarzana, CA: Third Line Press, 1999.

34. Thys-Jacobs, S., P. Starkey, D. Bernstein, et al. "Calcium Carbonate and the Premenstrual Syndrome: Effects on Premenstrual and Menstrual Symptoms. Premenstrual Syndrome Study Group." *Am J Obstet Gynecol* 179(2) (Aug 1998): 444–452.

35. Benton, D., J. Haller, J. Fordy. "Vitamin Supplementation for 1 Year Improves Mood." *Neuropsychobiology* 32(2) (1995):98–105.

36. Coppen, A., J. Bailey. "Enhancement of the Antidepressant Action of Fluoxetine by Folic Acid: A Randomised, Placebo Controlled Trial." *J Affect Disord* 60(2) (Nov 2000):121–130. Bell, I. R., J. Edman, F. D. Morrow, et al. "Vitamin B_1, B_2, and B_6 Augmentation of Tricyclic Antidepressant Treatment in Geriatric Depression with Cognitive Dysfunction." *J Am Coll Nutr* 11(2) (Apr 1992):159–163.

37. Fava, M., J. S. Borus, J. E. Alpert, et al. "Folate, Vitamin B_{12}, and Homocysteine in Major Depressive Disorder." *Am J Psychiatry* 154(3) (Mar 1997):426–428.

38. Hoffer, A., J. Prousky. *Naturopathic Nutrition: A Guide to Nutrient-Rich Food and Nutritional Supplements for Optimum Health.* Toronto, ON: CCNM Press, 2006.

39. Ibid.

40. Hoffer A, A. W. Saul, H. D. Foster. *Niacin: The Real Story.* Laguna Beach, CA: Basic Health Publications, 2011.

41. Werbach, M. R., J. Moss. *Textbook of Nutritional Medicine.* Tarzana, CA: Third Line Press, 1999.

42. Dean, C. *Hormone Balance.* Avon, Massachusettes: Adams Media, 2005.

43. Werbach, M. R., J. Moss. *Textbook of Nutritional Medicine.* Tarzana, CA: Third Line Press, 1999.

44. Dean, C. *Hormone Balance.* Avon, Massachusettes: Adams Media, 2005.

45. Benjamin, J., J. Levine, M. Fux, et al. "Double-Blind, Placebo-Controlled, Crossover Trial of Inositol Treatment for Panic Disorder." *Am J Psychiatry* 152(7) (Jul 1995):1084–1086. Fux, M., J. Levine, A. Aviv, et al. "Inositol Treatment of Obsessive-Compulsive Disorder." *Am J Psychiatry* 153(9) (Sep 1996):1219–1221. Levine, J., Y. Barak, M. Gonzalves, et al. "Double-Blind, Controlled Trial of Inositol Treatment of Depression." *Am J Psychiatry* 152(5) (May 1995):792–794.

46. Palatnik, A., K. Frolov, M. Fux, et al. "Double-Blind, Controlled, Crossover Trial of Inositol Versus Fluvoxamine for the Treatment of Panic Disorder." *J Clin Psychopharmacol* 21(3) (Jun 2001):335–9.

47. Benton, D., R. Cook. "The Impact of Selenium Supplementation on Mood." *Biol Psychiatry* 29(11) (Jun 1, 1991):1092–1098.

48. Hoffer A, A. W. Saul, H. D. Foster. *Niacin: The Real Story.* Laguna Beach, CA: Basic Health Publications, 2011.

49. Ibid.

50. Ibid.

51. Stewart, W. F., R. B. Lipton, D. D. Celentano, et al. "Prevalence of Migraine Headache in the United States." *JAMA* 267(1) (1992):64–69.

52. Spigt, M. G., E. C. Kuijper, C. P. Schayck, et al. "Increasing the Daily Water Intake for the Prophylactic Treatment of Headache: A Pilot Trial." *Eur J Neurol* 12(9) (Sep 2005):715–718.

53. van Dusseldorp, M., M. B. Katan. "Headache Caused by Caffeine Withdrawal among Moderate Coffee Drinkers Switched from Ordinary to Decaffeinated Coffee: A 12 Week Double Blind Trial." *Brit Med J* 300(6739) (Jun 16, 1990):1558–1559. James, J. E. "Acute and Chronic Effects of Caffeine on Performance, Mood, Headache, and Sleep." *Neuropsychobiology* 38(1) (1998): 32–41.

54. Facchinetti, F., G. Sances, P. Borella, et al. "Magnesium Prophylaxis of Menstrual Migraine: Effects on Intracellular Magnesium." *Headache* 31(5) (May 1991):298–301.

55. Schoenen, J., J. Jacquy, M. Lenaerts. "Effectiveness of High-Dose Riboflavin in Migraine Prophylaxis. A Randomized Controlled Trial." *Neurology* 50(2) (Feb 1998):466–470.

56. Hoffer, A., J. Prousky. *Naturopathic Nutrition: A Guide to Nutrient-Rich Food and Nutritional Supplements for Optimum Health*. Toronto, ON: CCNM Press, 2006.

57. Werbach, M. R., J. Moss. *Textbook of Nutritional Medicine*. Tarzana, CA: Third Line Press, 1999.

58. U. S. Department of Health and Human Services. National Institutes of Health. National Heart Lung and Blood Institute. "What Are the Signs and Symptoms of Iron-Deficiency Anemia?" http://www.nhlbi.nih.gov/health/health-topics/topics/ida/signs.html. (accessed October 2011).

59. U. S. Department of Health and Human Services. National Institutes of Health. National Heart Lung and Blood Institute. "Who Is at Risk for Iron-Deficiency Anemia?" http://www.nhlbi.nih.gov/health/health-topics/topics/ida/atrisk.html. (accessed October 2011). Looker, A. C., P. R. Dallman, M. D. Carroll, et al. "Prevalence of Iron Deficiency in the United States." *JAMA* 277(12) (1997):973–976.59.

60. Cheraskin, E., W. M. Ringsdorf Jr., F. H. Medford. "Daily Vitamin C Consumption and Fatigability." *J Am Geriatr Soc* 24(3) (Mar 1976):136–137.

61. Werbach, M. R., J. Moss. *Textbook of Nutritional Medicine*. Tarzana, CA: Third Line Press, 1999. Heap, L. C., T. J. Peters, S. Wessely. "Vitamin B Status in Patients with Chronic Fatigue Syndrome." *J R Soc Med* 92(4) (Apr 1999): 183–185.

62. Cox, I. M., M. J. Campbell, D. Dowson. "Red Blood Cell Magnesium and Chronic Fatigue Syndrome." *Lancet* 337(8744) (Mar 30, 1991):757–760.

63. Werbach, M. R., J. Moss. *Textbook of Nutritional Medicine*. Tarzana, CA: Third Line Press, 1999. Werbach, M. R. "Nutritional Strategies for Treating Chronic Fatigue Syndrome." *Altern Med Rev* 5(2) (Apr 2000):93–108.

64. Sin, C. W., J. S. Ho, J. W. Chung. "Systematic Review on the Effectiveness of

Caffeine Abstinence on the Quality of Sleep." *J Clin Nurs* 18(1) (Jan 2009):13–21. James, J. E. "Acute and Chronic Effects of Caffeine on Performance, Mood, Headache, and Sleep." *Neuropsychobiology* 38(1) (1998):32–41.

65. Montgomery, P., J. Dennis. "Physical Exercise for Sleep Problems in Adults Aged 60+." *Cochrane Database Syst Rev* 4 (2002):CD003404.

66. Depoortere, H., D. Françon, J. Llopis. "Effects of a Magnesium-Deficient Diet on Sleep Organization in Rats." *Neuropsychobiology* 27(4) (1993):237–245.

67. Kryger, M. H., K. Otake, J. Foerster. "Low Body Stores of Iron and Restless Legs Syndrome: A Correctable Cause of Insomnia in Adolescents and Teenagers." *Sleep Med* 3(2) (Mar 2002):127–132. Prevention Health Books. *Prevention's Best Vitamin Cures: The Ultimate Compendium of Vitamin and Mineral Cures with More than 500 Remedies for Whatever Ails You!*. New York: Rodale; St. Martin's Paperbacks, 2000.

68. Buscemi, N., B. Vandermeer, N. Hooton, et al. "Efficacy and Safety of Exogenous Melatonin for Secondary Sleep Disorders and Sleep Disorders Accompanying Sleep Restriction: Meta-analysis." *Brit Med J* 332(7538) (Feb 18, 2006):385–393.

69. Saul, A. W. *Doctor Yourself: Natural Healing That Works*. Laguna Beach, CA: Basic Health Publications, 2003.

70. Ibid.

71. Hoffer, A., A. W. Saul. *Orthomolecular Medicine for Everyone: Megavitamin Therapeutics for Families and Physicians*. Laguna Beach, CA: Basic Health Publications, 2008.

72. Saul, A. W. *Doctor Yourself: Natural Healing That Works*. Laguna Beach, CA: Basic Health Publications, 2003.

73. U. S. National Library of Medicine. National Institutes of Health. Medline Plus. "Heart Disease in Women." http://www.nlm.nih.gov/medlineplus/heartdiseaseinwomen.html (accessed October 2011).

74. Ibid.

75. U. S. Department of Health and Human Services Office on Women's Health. http://www.womenshealth.gov/publications/our-publications/fact-sheet/heart-disease.cfm#a (accessed October 2011).

76. Stampfer, M. J., C. H. Hennekens, J. E. Manson, et al. "Vitamin E Consumption and the Risk of Coronary Disease in Women." *N Engl J Med* 328(20) (May 20, 1993):1444–1449.

77. Osganian, S. K., M. J. Stampfer, E. Rimm, et al. "Vitamin C and Risk of Coronary Heart Disease in Women." *J Am Coll Cardiol* 42(2) (Jul 16, 2003):246–252.

78. Alderman, J. D., R. C. Pasternak, F. M. Sacks, et al. "Effect of a Modified, Well-Tolerated Niacin Regimen on Serum Total Cholesterol, High Density Lipoprotein Cholesterol and the Cholesterol to High Density Lipoprotein Ratio." *Am J Cardiol* 64(12) (Oct 1, 1989):725–729.

79. Malik, S., M. L. Kashyap. "Niacin, Lipids, and Heart Disease." *Curr Cardiol Rep* 5(6) (Nov 2003):470–476.

80. Orthomolecular Medicine News Service. "Way Too Many Prescriptions." August 11, 2008. http://www.orthomolecular.org/resources/omns/v04n07.shtml. (accessed October 2011).

81. Saul, A. W. *Fire Your Doctor: How to be Independently Healthy.* Laguna Beach, CA: Basic Health Publications, 2005.

82. Kaufman, W. *The Common Form of Joint Dysfunction.* Brattleboro, VT: E.L. Hildreth and Co., 1949. Pages 20–29 available online at: http://www.DoctorYourself.com/kaufman5.html. (accessed October 2011).

CHAPTER 6. PROBLEMS WITH THE PILL AND OTHER FORMS OF HORMONAL BIRTH CONTROL

1. Robinson, J. C., S. Plichta, C. S. Weisman, et al. "Dysmenorrhea and Use of Oral Contraceptives in Adolescent Women Attending a Family Planning Clinic." *Am J Obstet Gynecol* 166(2) (Feb 1992):578–583.

2. Arowojolu, A. O., M. F. Gallo, L. M. Lopez, et al. "Combined Oral Contraceptive Pills for Treatment of Acne." *Cochrane Database Syst Rev* 3 (2009): CD004425.

3. Vercellini, P., G. Frontino, O. De Giorgi, et al. "Continuous Use of an Oral Contraceptive for Endometriosis-Associated Recurrent Dysmenorrhea that Does Not Respond to a Cyclic Pill Regimen." *Fertil Steril* 80(3) (Sep 2003):560–563.

4. Schlesselman, J. J. "Net Effect of Oral Contraceptive Use on the Risk of Cancer in Women in the United States." *Obstet Gynecol* 85(5 Pt 1) (May 1995): 793–801.

5. Piccinio, L., W. Mosher. "Trends in Contraceptive Use in the United States: 1982–1995." *Fam Plann Perspect* 30(1) (Jan-Feb 1998):4–10, 46. Mosher, W.D., G. M. Martinez, A. Chandra, et al. "Use of Contraception and Use of Family Planning Services in the United States: 1982–2002." *Adv Data* 350 (Dec 10, 2004):1–36.

6. Ibid.

7. Westhoff, C. "Contraception at Age 35 Years and Older." *Clin Obstet Gynecol* 41(4) (Dec 1998):951–957.

8. RxList: The Internet Drug Index. www.rxlist.com. (accessed October 2011).

9. Ibid.

10. Roberts, S. C., L. M. Gosling, V. Carter, et al. "MHC-Correlated Odour Preferences in Humans and the Use of Oral Contraceptives." *Proc R Soc B* 275 (2008):2715–2722.

11. Roberts, S. C., L. M. Gosling, V. Carter, et al. "MHC-Correlated Odour Preferences in Humans and the Use of Oral Contraceptives." *Proc R Soc B* 275 (2008):2715–2722. Wedekind, C., T. Seebeck, F. Bettens, et al. "MHC-Depend-

ent Mate Preferences in Humans." *Proc Biol Sci* 260(1359) (Jun 22, 1995): 245–249.

12. Seppo Kuukasjärvi, C. J. P. Eriksson, E. Koskela, et al. "Attractiveness of Women's Body Odors over the Menstrual Cycle: The Role of Oral Contraceptives and Receiver Sex." *Behav Ecol* 15(4) (2004):579–584.

13. Singh, D., M. Bronstad. "Female Body Odour is a Potential Cue to Ovulation." *Proc Biol Sci* 268(1469) (Apr 22, 2001):797–801.

14. Alvergne, A., V. Lummaa. "Does the contraceptive pill alter mate choice in humans?" *Trends Ecol Evol* 25(3) (2009):171–179.

15. Ibid.

16. Ibid.

17. Brinton, L., J. Daling, J. Liff, et al. "Oral Contraceptives and Breast Cancer Risk among Younger Women." *J Natl Cancer Inst* 87(11) (Jun 7, 1995):827–835. Burkman R., J. J. Schlesselman, M. Zieman. "Safety Concerns and Health Benefits Associated with Oral Contraception." *Am J Obstet Gynecol* 190(4 Suppl) (Apr 2004):S5-S22.

18. Brinton, L., J. Daling, J. Liff, et al. "Oral Contraceptives and Breast Cancer Risk among Younger Women." *J Natl Cancer Inst* 87(11) (Jun 7, 1995):827–835.

19. Brinton, L., J. Daling, J. Liff, et al. "Oral Contraceptives and Breast Cancer Risk among Younger Women." *J Natl Cancer Inst* 87(11) (Jun 7, 1995):827–835. Calle, E. E., C. W. Heath Jr., H. L. Miracle-McMahill, et al. "Breast Cancer and Hormonal Contraceptives:Collaborative Reanalysis of Individual Data on 53, 297 Women with Breast Cancer and 100, 239 Women without Breast Cancer from 54 Epidemiological Studies." *Lancet* 347(9017) (Jun 22, 1996):1713–1727.

20. Brinton, L., J. Daling, J. Liff, et al. "Oral Contraceptives and Breast Cancer Risk among Younger Women." *J Natl Cancer Inst* 87(11) (Jun 7, 1995):827–835.

21. Calle, E. E., C. W. Heath Jr., H. L. Miracle-McMahill, et al. "Breast Cancer and Hormonal Contraceptives:Collaborative Reanalysis of Individual Data on 53, 297 Women with Breast Cancer and 100, 239 Women without Breast Cancer from 54 Epidemiological Studies." *Lancet* 347(9017) (Jun 22, 1996):1713–1727.

22. Schlesselman, J. J. "Net Effect of Oral Contraceptive Use on the Risk of Cancer in Women in the United States." *Obstet Gynecol* 85(5 Pt 1) (May 1995):793–801. Moreno, V., F. X. Bosch, N. Muñoz, et al. "Effect of Oral Contraceptives on Risk of Cervical Cancer in Women with Human Papillomavirus Infection: The IARC Multicentric Case-Control Study." *Lancet* 359(9312) (Mar 30, 2002):1085–1092.

23. Moreno, V., F. X. Bosch, N. Muñoz, et al. "Effect of Oral Contraceptives on Risk of Cervical Cancer in Women with Human Papillomavirus Infection: The IARC Multicentric Case-Control Study." *Lancet* 359(9312) (Mar 30, 2002):1085–1092.

24. Ibid.

25. Ibid.

26. Smith, J. S., J. Green, A. B. de Gonzalez, et al. "Cervical Cancer and Use of Hormonal Contraceptives: A Systematic Review." *Lancet* 361(9364) (Apr 5, 2003):1159–1167.

27. Forman, D., T. J. Vincent, R. Doll. "Cancer of the Liver and the Use of Oral Contraceptives." *Brit Med J (Clin Res Ed)* 292(6532) (May 24, 1986):1357–1361. Hsing, A. W., R. N. Hoover, J. K. McLaughlin, et al. "Oral Contraceptives and Primary Liver Cancer among Young Women." *Cancer Causes Control* 3(1) (Jan 1992):43–48. Palmer, J. R., L. Rosenberg, D. W. Kaufman, et al. "Oral Contraceptive Use and Liver Cancer." *Am J Epidemiol* 130(5) (1989):878–882.

28. Brinton, L., J. Daling, J. Liff, et al. "Oral Contraceptives and Breast Cancer Risk among Younger Women." *J Natl Cancer Inst* 87(11) (Jun 7, 1995):827–835. Tanis, B. C., M. A. A. J. van den Bosch, J. M. Kemmeren, et al. "Oral Contraceptives and the Risk of Myocardial Infarction." *New Eng J Med* 345(25) (Dec 20, 2001):1787–1793. Poulter, N. R, C.L. Chang, T. M. M. Farley, et al. "Ischaemic Stroke and Combined Oral Contraceptives: Results of an International, Multicentre, Case-Control Study." *Lancet* 348(9026) (Aug 24, 1996):498–505. Heinemann, L. A. J, M. A. Lewis, M. Thorogood, et al. "Case-Control Study of Oral Contraceptives and Risk of Thromboembolic Stroke: Results from International Study on Oral Contraceptives and Health of Young Women." *Brit Med J* 315:7121 (1997): 1502–1504. Kemmeren, J. M., A. Algra, D. E. Grobbee. "Third Generation Oral Contraceptives and Risk of Venous Thrombosis: Meta Analysis." *Brit Med J* 323(7305) (Jul 21, 2001):131–134.

29. Stadel, B. V. "Oral Contraceptives and Cardiovascular Disease. (Second of Two Parts)." *New Eng J Med* 305(12) (1981):672–677. Croft, P., P. Hannaford. "Risk Factors for Acute Myocardial Infarction in Women: Evidence from the Royal College of General Practitioners' Oral Contraception Study." *Brit Med J* 298(6667) (Jan 21, 1989):165–168.

30. Pymar, H. C., M. D. Creinin. "The Risks of Oral Contraceptive Pills." *Semin Reprod Med* 19(4) (Dec 2001). 305–312. Available online: http://www.medscape.com/viewarticle/421027 (accessed October 2011).

31. Schlesselman, J. J. "Net Effect of Oral Contraceptive Use on the Risk of Cancer in Women in the United States." *Obstet Gynecol* 85(5 Pt 1) (May 1995): 793–801.

32. Mosher, W.D., G. M. Martinez, A. Chandra, et al. "Use of Contraception and Use of Family Planning Services in the United States: 1982–2002." *Adv Data* 350 (Dec 10, 2004):1–36.

33. Pymar, H. C., M. D. Creinin. "The Risks of Oral Contraceptive Pills." *Semin Reprod Med* 19(4) (Dec 2001). 305–312. Available online: http://www.medscape.com/viewarticle/421027 (accessed October 2011).

34. National Safety Council. "The Odds of Dying From . . ." http://www.nsc.org/news_resources/injury_and_death_statistics/Pages/TheOddsofDyingFrom.aspx. (accessed October 2011).

35. Gerstman, B., J. Piper, D. Tornita, et al. "Oral Contraceptive Estrogen Dose and the Risk of Deep Venous Thromboembolic Disease." *Am J Epidemiol* 133(1) (Jan 1991):32–37.

36. Thorneycroft, I. H., S. L. Cariati. "Ultra-Low-Dose Contraceptives: Are They Right for Your Patient?" *Medscape General Med* 3(4) (2001). http://www.medscape.com/viewarticle/408944. (accessed October 2011).

37. Ibid.

38. Meade, T. W., G. Greenberg, S. G. Thompson. "Progestogens and Cardiovascular Reactions Associated with Oral contraceptives and a Comparison of the Safety of 50- and 30-Microgram Oestrogen Preparations." *Brit Med J* 280(6224) (May 10, 1980):1157–61.

39. Cassidy, S. "Birth Control Patch Cases Being Settled and Sealed." Get Legal/Public. TheAttorneyStore.com. http://public.getlegal.com/articles/birth-control-patch-cases. (accessed October 2011).

40. Wynn, V. "Vitamins and Oral Contraceptive Use." *Lancet* 305(7906) (Mar 1975):561–564. Haas, E. M. "Nutrient Program for Oral Contraceptives." Healthy.net. HealthWorld Online. http://www.healthy.net/scr/Article.aspx?Id=1260. (accessed October 2011). Webb, J. L. "Nutritional Effects of Oral Contraceptive Use: A Review." *J Reprod Med* 25(4) (Oct 1980):150–156.

41. Dean, C. *Hormone Balance: A Woman's Guide to Restoring Health and Vitality.* Avon, MA: Adams Media, 2005.

42. Lussana, F., M. L. Zighetti, P. Bucciarelli, et al. "Blood Levels of Homocysteine, Folate, Vitamin B_6 and B_{12} in Women Using Oral Contraceptives Compared to Non-Users." *Thromb Res* 112(1–2) (2003):37–41.

43. Rinehart, J. F, and L. D. Greenberg. "Vitamin B_6 Deficiency in the Rhesus Monkey." *Am J Clin Nutr* 4 (Jul-Aug 1956):318–328. Robinson, K., K. Arheart, H. Refsum, et al. "Low Circulating Folate and Vitamin B_6 Concentrations: Risk Factors for Stroke, Peripheral Vascular disease, and Coronary Artery Disease." *Circulation* 97(5) (Feb 10, 1998):437–443.

44. Lussana, F., M. L. Zighetti, P. Bucciarelli, et al. "Blood Levels of Homocysteine, Folate, Vitamin B_6 and B_{12} in Women Using Oral Contraceptives Compared to Non-Users." *Thromb Res* 112(1–2) (2003):37–41. Hron, G., R. Lombardi, S. Eichinger, et al. "Low Vitamin B_6 Levels and the Risk of Recurrent Venous Thromboembolism." *Haematologica* 92(9) (Sep2007):1250–1253.

45. Zhang, S. M., W. C. Willett, J. Selhub, et al. "Plasma Folate, Vitamin B6, Vitamin B12, Homocysteine, and Risk of Breast Cancer." *J Natl Cancer Inst* 95(5) (Mar 5, 2003):373–380.

46. Lajous, M., E. Lazcano-Ponce, M. Hernandez-Avila, et al. "Folate, Vitamin B_6, and Vitamin B_{12} Intake and the Risk of Breast Cancer among Mexican Women." *Cancer Epidem Biomar* 15(3) (Mar 2006):443–448.

47. American Heart Association. "Homocysteine, Folic Acid and Cardiovascular Disease." http://www.heart.org/HEARTORG/GettingHealthy/NutritionCenter/

Homocysteine-Folic-Acid-and-Cardiovascular-Disease_UCM_305997_Article
.jsp#.TrAHPHK9JOw. (accessed October 2011).

48. Vermeulen, E. G., C. D. Stehouwer, J. W. Twisk, et al. "Effect of Homocysteine-Lowering Treatment with Folic Acid Plus Vitamin B_6 on Progression of Subclinical Atherosclerosis: A Randomised, Placebo-Controlled Trial." *Lancet* 355(9203) (Feb 12, 2000):517–522. Brattström L., B. Israelsson, B. Norrving, et al. "Impaired Homocysteine Metabolism in Early-Onset Cerebral and Peripheral Occlusive Arterial Disease. Effects of Pyridoxine and Folic Acid Treatment." *Atherosclerosis* 81(1) (Feb 1990):51–60. van den Berg, M., D. G. Franken, G. H. Boers, et al. "Combined Vitamin B_6 Plus Folic Acid Therapy in Young patients with Arteriosclerosis and Hyperhomocysteinemia." *J Vas Surg* 20(6) (Dec 1994):933–940.

49. Office of Dietary Supplements. National Institute of Health. "Dietary Supplement Fact Sheet: Vitamin B_6." http://ods.od.nih.gov/factsheets/vitaminb6.asp. (accessed October 2011).

50. Morris, M. S., M .F. Picciano, P. F. Jacques, et al. "Plasma Pyridoxal 5'-Phosphate in the US Population: The National Health and Nutrition Examination Survey, 2003–2004." *Am J Clin Nutr* 87(5) (May 2008):1446–1454.

51. Ibid.

52. Ibid.

53. American Heart Association. "Homocysteine, Folic Acid and Cardiovascular Disease." http://www.heart.org/HEARTORG/GettingHealthy/NutritionCenter/Homocysteine-Folic-Acid-and-Cardiovascular-Disease_UCM_305997_Article
.jsp#.TrAHPHK9JOw. (accessed October 2011).

54. den Heijer, M., I. A. Brouwer, G. M. Bos, et al. "Vitamin Supplementation Reduces Blood Homocysteine Levels: A Controlled Trial in Patients with Venous Thrombosis and Healthy Volunteers." *Arterioscler Thromb Vasc Biol* 18(3) (Mar 1998):356–361. Brouwer, I. A., M. van Dusseldorp, C. M. G. Thomas, et al. "Low-Dose Folic Acid Supplementation Decreases Plasma Homocysteine Concentrations: A Randomised Trial." *Indian Heart J* 52(Suppl 7) (Nov-Dec 2000): S53–58.

55. Vermeulen, E. G., C. D. Stehouwer, J. W. Twisk, et al. "Effect of Homocysteine-Lowering Treatment with Folic Acid Plus Vitamin B_6 on Progression of Subclinical Atherosclerosis: A Randomised, Placebo-Controlled Trial." *Lancet* 355(9203) (Feb 12, 2000):517–522.

56. Guo, H., J. D. Lee, H. Uzui, et al. "Effects of Folic Acid and Magnesium on the Production of Homocysteine-Induced Extracellular Matrix Metalloproteinase-2 in Cultured Rat Vascular Smooth Muscle Cells." *Circ J* 70(1) (Jan 2006):141–146.

57. Winston, F. "Oral Contraceptives, Pyridoxine, and Depression." *Am J Psychiatry* 130(11) (Nov 1973):1217–1221.

58. Challem, J. *The Food Mood Solution.* Hoboken, NJ: John Wiley & Sons, 2007.

59. Ibid.

60. Saul, A. W. *Fire Your Doctor: How to be Independently Healthy*. Laguna Beach, CA: Basic Health Publications, 2005. Pauling, L. *How to Live Longer and Feel Better*. Corvallis, OR: Oregon State University Press, 2006.

61. Cohen, M., A. Bendich. "Safety of Pyridoxine—A Review of Human and Animal Studies." *Toxicol Lett* 32(2–3) (Dec 1986):129–139. Gaby, A. R. "'Safe Upper Levels' for Nutritional Supplements: One Giant Step Backward." *J Orthomolecular Med* 18(3–4) (2003):126–130.

62. Pauling, L. *How to Live Longer and Feel Better*. Corvallis, OR: Oregon State University Press, 2006.

63. Ibid.

64. Hoffer, A., A. W. Saul. *Orthomolecular Medicine for Everyone: Megavitamin Therapeutics for Families and Physicians*. Laguna Beach, CA: Basic Health Publications, 2008.

65. Pauling, L. *How to Live Longer and Feel Better*. Corvallis, OR: Oregon State University Press, 2006. Hoffer, A., J. Prousky. *Naturopathic Nutrition: A Guide to Nutrient-Rich Food and Nutritional Supplements for Optimum Health*. Toronto, ON: CCNM Press, 2006.

66. Bronstein A.C., D.A. Spyker, L.R, Cantilena Jr, et al. "2009 Annual Report of the American Association of Poison Control Centers' National Poison Data System (NPDS): 27th Annual Report." *Clin Toxicol* 48(10) (Dec 2010):979–1178. Available at: http://www.aapcc.org/dnn/Portals/0/2009%AR.pdf. (accessed October 2011).

67. Pauling, L. *How to Live Longer and Feel Better*. Corvallis, OR: Oregon State University Press, 2006.

68. Ibid.

69. Ford, E. S., A. H. Mokdad. "Dietary Magnesium Intake in a National Sample of US Adults." *J Nutr* 133(9) (Sep 2003):2879–2882. King, D. E., A. G. Mainous 3rd, M. E. Geesey, et al. "Dietary Magnesium and C-Reactive Protein Levels." *J Am Coll Nutr* 24(3) (Jun 2005):166–171.

70. Institute of Medicine, Food and Nutrition Board. *Dietary Reference Intakes for Vitamin A, Vitamin K, Arsenic, Boron, Chromium, Copper, Iodine, Iron, Manganese, Molybdenum, Nickel, Silicon, Vanadium, and Zinc*. Washington, DC: National Academies Press, 2001.

71. Bogden, J. D., J. M. Oleske, E. M. Munves, et al. "Zinc and Immunocompetence in the Elderly: Baseline Data on Zinc Nutriture and Immunity in Unsupplemented Subjects." *Amer J Clin Nutr* 46(1) (Jul 1987):101–109.

72. Hoffer, A., A. W. Saul. *Orthomolecular Medicine for Everyone: Megavitamin Therapeutics for Families and Physicians*. Laguna Beach, CA: Basic Health Publications, 2008.

73. Office of Dietary Supplements. National Institute of Health. "Dietary Supple-

ment Fact Sheet: Zinc." http://ods.od.nih.gov/factsheets/Zinc. (accessed October 2011).

CHAPTER 7. URINARY TRACT INFECTIONS

1. Foxman, B. "Epidemiology of Urinary Tract Infections: Incidence, Morbidity, and Economic Costs." *Am J Med* 113(Suppl 1A) (Jul 8, 2002):5S-13S.

2. Foxman, B. "Epidemiology of Urinary Tract Infections: Incidence, Morbidity, and Economic Costs." *Am J Med* 113(Suppl 1A) (Jul 8, 2002):5S-13S. Griebling, T. L. "Urologic Diseases in America Project: Trends in Resource Use for Urinary Tract Infections in Women." *J Urol* 173(4) (Apr 2005):1281-1287.

3. Franco, A. V. "Recurrent Urinary Tract Infections." *Best Pract Res Clin Obstet Gynaecol* 19(6) (Dec 2005):861-73.

4. Griebling, T. L. "Urologic Diseases in America Project: Trends in Resource Use for Urinary Tract Infections in Women." *J Urol* 173(4) (Apr 2005):1281-1287.

5. Hooton, T. M., R. Besser, B. Foxman, et al. "Acute Uncomplicated Cystitis in an Era of Increasing Antibiotic Resistance: A Proposed Approach to Empirical Therapy." *Clin Infect Dis* 39(1) (Jul 1, 2004):75-80.

6. U.S. Department of Health and Human Services. Office on Women's Health. Womenshealth.gov. "Urinary Tract Infection Fact Sheet." http://womenshealth .gov/publications/our-publications/fact-sheet/urinary-tract-infection.cfm. (accessed October 2011).

7. Ibid.

8. Foxman, B. "Epidemiology of Urinary Tract Infections: Incidence, Morbidity, and Economic Costs." *Am J Med* 113(Suppl 1A) (Jul 8, 2002):5S-13S.

9. Familydoctor.org Editorial Staff. "Urinary Tract Infections." FamilyDoctor.org. http://familydoctor.org/familydoctor/en/diseases-conditions/urinary-tract-infec-tions.html. (accessed October 2011).

10. Foxman, B. "Epidemiology of Urinary Tract Infections: Incidence, Morbidity, and Economic Costs." *Am J Med* 113(Suppl 1A) (Jul 8, 2002):5S-13S. U.S. Department of Health and Human Services. Office on Women's Health. Women-shealth.gov. "Urinary Tract Infection Fact Sheet." http://womenshealth.gov/pub-lications/our-publications/fact-sheet/urinary-tract-infection.cfm. (accessed October 2011). Fihn, S. D., R. H. Latham, P Roberts, et al. "Association between Diaphragm Use and Urinary Tract Infection." *JAMA* 254(2) (Jul 12, 1985):240-245.

11. Peterson, J., S. Kaul, M. Khashab, et al. "Identification and Pretherapy Sus-ceptibility of Pathogens in Patients with Complicated Urinary Tract Infection or Acute Pyelonephritis Enrolled in a Clinical Study in the United States from November 2004 through April 2006." *Clin Ther* 29(10) (Oct 2007):2215-2221. Zhanel, G. G., T. L. Hisanaga, N. M. Laing, et al. "Antibiotic Resistance in Out-patient Urinary Isolates: Final Results from the North American Urinary Tract Infection Collaborative Alliance (NAUTICA)." *Int J Antimicrob Agents* 26(5)

(Nov 2005):380–388. Karlowsky, J. A., D. J. Hoban, M. R. Decorby, et al. "Fluoroquinolone-Resistant Urinary Isolates of Escherichia coli from Outpatients Are Frequently Multidrug Resistant: Results from the North American Urinary Tract Infection Collaborative Alliance-Quinolone Resistance Study." *Antimicrob Agents Chemother* 50(6) (Jun 2006):2251–2254. Hames, L., and C. E. Rice. "Antimicrobial Resistance of Urinary Tract Isolates in Acute Uncomplicated Cystitis among College-Aged Women: Choosing a First-Line Therapy." *J Am Coll Health* 56(2) (Sep-Oct 2007):153–156. Gupta, K., T. M. Hooton, and W. E. Stamm. "Increasing Antimicrobial Resistance and the Management of Uncomplicated Community-Acquired Urinary Tract Infections." *Ann Intern Med* 135(1) (Jul 3, 2001):41–50. Aypak, C., A. Altunsoy, N. Düzgün. "Empiric Antibiotic Therapy in Acute Uncomplicated Urinary Tract Infections and Fluoroquinolone Resistance: A Prospective Observational Study." *Ann Clin Microbiol Antimicrob* 8 (Oct 24, 2009):27. Kurutepe, S., S. Surucuoglu, C. Sezgin, et al. "Increasing Antimicrobial Resistance in *Escherichia coli* Isolates from Community-Acquired Urinary Tract Infections during 1998–2003 in Manisa, Turkey." *Jpn J Infect Dis* 58(3) (Jun 2005):159–161. Lee, S. J., S. D. Lee, I. R. Cho, et al. "Antimicrobial Susceptibility of Uropathogens Causing Acute Uncomplicated Cystitis in Female Outpatients in South Korea: A Multicentre Study in 2002." *Inter J Antimicrob Agents* 24(Suppl 1) (Sep 2004):S61-S64.

12. Hames, L., and C. E. Rice. "Antimicrobial Resistance of Urinary Tract Isolates in Acute Uncomplicated Cystitis among College-Aged Women: Choosing a First-Line Therapy." *J Am Coll Health* 56(2) (Sep-Oct 2007):153–156. Gupta, K., T. M. Hooton, P. L. Roberts, et al. "Emergence of Fluoroquinolone-Resistant E. Coli after Treatment of Acute Uncomplicated Cystitis." *Abstr Intersci Conf Antimicrob Agents Chemother* 43(abstract no. L-265) (Sep 14–17, 2003).

13. Foxman, B. "Recurring Urinary Tract Infection: Incidence and Risk Factors." *Am J Public Health* 80(3) (Mar 1990):331–333.

14. Fihn, S. "Acute Uncomplicated Urinary Tract Infection in Women." *N Engl J Med* 349 (Jul 17, 2003):259–266.

15. Brown, P. D., A. Freeman, B. Foxman. "Prevalence and Predictors of Trimethoprim-Sulfamethoxazole Resistance among Uropathogenic Escherichia Coli Isolates in Michigan." *Clin Infect Dis* 34(8) (Apr 15, 2002):1061–1066.

16. RxList. The Internet Drug Index. Information for trimethoprim/sulfamethoxazole, nitrofurantoin, ampicillin, and fluoroquinolone. http://www.rxlist.com/script/main/hp.asp. (accessed November 2011).

17. United States Department of Health and Human Services. United States Food and Drug Administration (FDA). "Information for Healthcare Professionals: Fluoroquinolone Antimicrobial Drugs [ciprofloxacin (marketed as Cipro and generic ciprofloxacin), ciprofloxacin extended-release (marketed as Cipro XR and Proquin XR), gemifloxacin (marketed as Factive), levofloxacin (marketed as Levaquin), moxifloxacin (marketed as Avelox), norfloxacin (marketed as Noroxin), and ofloxacin (marketed as Floxin)]." http://www.fda.gov/Drugs/DrugSafety/PostmarketDrugSafetyInformationforPatientsandProviders/ucm126085.htm. (accessed

November 2011). Physician's Desk Reference. Cipro XR Concise Monograph. http://www.pdr.net/drugpages/concisemonograph.aspx?concise=2010 (accessed November 2011).

18. Reid, G. "Probiotics to Prevent the Need for, and Augment the Use of, Antibiotics." *Can J Infect Dis Med Microbiol* 17(5) (Sep-Oct 2006):291–295.

19. Prevention Health Books. *Prevention's Best Vitamin Cures: The Ultimate Compendium of Vitamin and Mineral Cures with More than 500 Remedies for Whatever Ails You!*. New York: Rodale; St. Martin's Paperbacks, 2000.

20. PRN Newswire. "Americans Relate Water To Well-Being, But Most Don't Get Their Fill; Survey Shows 33 Percent of What Americans Drink Can Cause Dehydration." (May 30, 2000). http://www.thefreelibrary.com/Americans+Relate+Water+To+Well-Being,+But+Most+Don%27t+Get+Their+Fill%3B...-a062446342. (accessed October 2011).

21. Balch, J. F., P. A. Balch. *Prescriptions for Natural Healing.* New York, NY: Avery Publishing Group, 1990.

22. Jepson, R. G., L. Mihaljevic, J. Craig. "Cranberries for Preventing Urinary Tract Infections." *Cochrane DB Syst Rev* 2 (2004): CD001321. Jepson, R. G., J. Craig. "Cranberries for Preventing Urinary Tract Infections." Update. *Cochrane DB Syst Rev* 1 (2008): CD001321. Kontiokari, T., K. Sundqvist, M. Nuutinen, et al. "Randomised Trial of Cranberry-Lingonberry Juice and Lactobacillus GG Drink for the Prevention of Urinary Tract Infections in Women." *Brit Med J* 322(7302) (Jun 30, 2001):1571. Stothers, L. "A Randomized Trial to Evaluate Effectiveness and Cost Effectiveness of Naturopathic Cranberry Products as Prophylaxis against Urinary Tract Infection in Women." *Can J Urol* 9(3) (Jun 2002):1558–1562.

23. Zafriri, D., I. Ofek, R. Adar, et al. "Inhibitory Activity of Cranberry Juice on Adherence of Type 1 and Type P Fimbriated Escherichia Coli to Eucaryotic Cells." *Antimicrob Agents Chemother* 33(1) (Jan 1989):92–98. Ofek, I., J. Goldhar, D. Zafriri, et al. "Anti-Escherichia Coli Adhesin Activity of Cranberry and Blueberry Juices." *N Engl J Med* 324(22) (May 30, 1991):1599. Schmidt, D. R., A. E. Sobota. "An Examination of the Anti-Adherence Activity of Cranberry Juice on Urinary and Nonurinary Bacterial Isolates." *Microbios* 55(224–225) (1988): 173–181.

24. Berkson, D. L. *Natural Answers for Women's Health Questions.* New York, NY: Simon & Schuster, 2002.

25. Raz, R., W. E. Stamm. "A Controlled Trial of Intravaginal Estriol in Postmenopausal Women with Recurrent Urinary Tract Infections." *N Engl J Med* 329(11) (Sep 9, 1993):753–756. Perrotta, C., M. Aznar, R. Mejia, et al. "Oestrogens for Preventing Recurrent Urinary Tract Infection in Postmenopausal Women." *Cochrane DB Syst Rev* 2 (Apr 16, 2008): CD005131.

26. MedicineNet.com "estrogens (synthetic)-vaginal cream. Side Effects." http://www.medicinenet.com/estrogens_synthetic-vaginal_cream/page2.htm. (accessed October 2011).

27. Werbach, M. R., J. Moss. *Textbook of Nutritional Medicine.* Tarzana, CA: Third Line Press, 1999.

28. Diplock, A. T. "Safety of Antioxidant Vitamins and Beta-Carotene." *Am J Clin Nutr* 62(6) (1995):1510S-1516S. Bendich, A. "The Safety of Beta-Carotene." *Nutr-Cancer* 11(4) (1988): 207–214.

29. Saul, A. W. *Doctor Yourself: Natural Healing That Works.* Laguna Beach, CA: Basic Health Publications, 2003.

30. Werbach, M. R., J. Moss. *Textbook of Nutritional Medicine.* Tarzana, CA: Third Line Press, 1999. Bendich, A. "Vitamin E and Immune Functions." *Basic Life Sci* 49 (1988):615–620. Meydani, S. N., M. P. Barklund, S. Liu, et al. "Vitamin E Supplementation Enhances Cell-Mediated Immunity in Healthy Elderly Subjects." *Am J Clin Nutr* 52(3) (Sep 1990):557–563.

31. Werbach, M. R., J. Moss. *Textbook of Nutritional Medicine.* Tarzana, CA: Third Line Press, 1999.

32. Ibid.

33. Hoffer, A., J. Prousky. *Naturopathic Nutrition: A Guide to Nutrient-Rich Food and Nutritional Supplements for Optimum Health.* Toronto, ON: CCNM Press, 2006.

34. American Cancer Society. "Learn About Cancer. Bladder Cancer." http://www.cancer.org/Cancer/BladderCancer/DetailedGuide/bladder-cancer-risk-factors. (accessed October 2011).

35. Lamm, D.L., D. R. Riggs, J. S. Shriver, et al. "Megadose Vitamins in Bladder Cancer: A Double-Blind Clinical Trial." *J Urol* 151(1) (Jan 1994):21–26.

36. Ibid.

37. Bronstein, A.C., D.A. Spyker, L. R., Cantilena Jr, et al. "2008 Annual Report of the American Association of Poison Control Centers' National Poison Data System (NPDS): 26th Annual Report." *Clin Toxicol* 47 (2009):911–1084. http://www.aapcc.org/dnn/Portals/0/2008annualreport.pdf. (accessed October 2011).

38. Bronstein, A. C., D. A. Spyker, L. R. Cantilena Jr, et al. "2009 Annual Report of the American Association of Poison Control Centers' National Poison Data System (NPDS): 27th Annual Report." *Clinical Toxicology* 48 (2010): 979–1178. http://www.aapcc.org/dnn/Portals/0/2009%20AR.pdf. (accessed October 2011).

39. Orthomolecular Medicine News Service. "Zero Deaths from Vitamins, Minerals, Amino Acids or Herbs. Poison Control Statistics Prove Supplements' Safety Yet Again." Jan 5, 2011. http://orthomolecular.org/resources/omns/v07n01.shtml. (accessed October 2011).

CHAPTER 8. ENDOMETRIOSIS

1. Stöppler, M. C., W. C. Shiel, Jr. "Endometriosis." MedicineNet.com. http://www.medicinenet.com/endometriosis/article.htm. (accessed October 2011).

2. U. S. National Library of Medicine. National Institutes of Health. Medline Plus. "Endometritis." http://www.nlm.nih.gov/medlineplus/ency/article/001484.htm. (accessed October 2011).

3. Rivlin, M. E. "Endometritis." Medscape Reference. WebMD. http://emedicine.medscape.com/article/254169-overview. (accessed October 2011).

4. Ness, R. B., D. E. Soper, R. L. Holley, et al. "Douching and Endometritis: Results from the PID Evaluation and Clinical Health (PEACH) Study." *Sex Transm Dis* 28(4) (Apr 2001):240–245.

5. Holzman, C., Leventhal, J. M., H. Qui, et al. "Factors Linked to Bacterial Vaginosis in Nonpregnant Women." *Am J Public Health.* 91(10) (Oct 2001):1664–1670.

6. Haggerty, C. L., S. L. Hillier, D. C. Bass, et al. "Bacterial Vaginosis and Anaerobic Bacteria are Associated with Endometritis." *Clin Infect Dis* 39(7) (Oct 1, 2004):990–995. Hillier, S. L. N. B. Kiviat, S. E. Hawes, et al. "Role of Bacterial Vaginosis-Associated Microorganisms in Endometritis." *Am J Obstet Gynecol* 175(2) (Aug 1996):435–441. Newton, E. R., T. J. Prihoda, R. S. Gibbs. "A Clinical and Microbiologic Analysis of Risk Factors for Puerperal Endometritis." *Obstet Gynecol* 75(3 Pt 1) (Mar 1990):402–406. Korn, A. P., G. Bolan, N. Padian, et al. "Plasma Cell Endometritis in Women with Symptomatic Bacterial Vaginosis." *Obstet Gynecol* 85(3) (Mar 1995):387–390.

7. Haggerty, C. L., S. L. Hillier, D. C. Bass, et al. "Bacterial Vaginosis and Anaerobic Bacteria are Associated with Endometritis." *Clin Infect Dis* 39(7) (Oct 1, 2004):990–995.

8. Grodstein, F., M. B. Goldman, D. W. Cramer. "Infertility in Women and Moderate Alcohol Use." *Am J Public Health* 84:9 (1994): 1429–1432.

9. Grodstein, F., M. B. Goldman, D. W. Cramer. "Endometriosis and Moderate Alcohol Use: Grodstein and Colleagues Respond." Letter. *Am J Public Health* 85(7) (Jul 1995):1021–1022.

10. Bérubé, S., S. Marcoux, R. Maheux. "Characteristics Related to the Prevalence of Minimal or Mild Endometriosis in Infertile Women. Canadian Collaborative Group on Endometriosis." *Epidemiology* 9(5) (Sep 1998):504–510. Grodstein, F., M. B. Goldman, L. Ryan, et al. "Relation of Female Infertility to Consumption of Caffeinated Beverages." *Am J Epidemiol* 137(12) (Jun 15, 1993):1353–1360.

11. Bérubé, S., S. Marcoux, R. Maheux. "Characteristics Related to the Prevalence of Minimal or Mild Endometriosis in Infertile Women. Canadian Collaborative Group on Endometriosis." *Epidemiology* 9(5) (Sep 1998):504–510.

12. Missmer, S. A., J. E. Chavarro, S. Malspeis, et al. "A Prospective Study of Dietary Fat Consumption and Endometriosis Risk." *Hum Reprod* 25(6) (Jun 2010):1528–1535.

13. Mayo Clinic Staff. "Endometriosis. Risk Factors." May Clinic. http://www.mayoclinic.com/health/endometriosis/DS00289/DSECTION=risk-factors. (accessed

October 2011). Cramer, D. W., S. A. Missmer. "The Epidemiology of Endometriosis." *Ann N Y Acad Sci* 955 (Mar 2002):11–22, discussion 34–36, 396–406. U.S. National Library of Medicine National Institutes of Health. "Endometriosis." http://www.ncbi.nlm.nih.gov/pubmedhealth/PMH0001913. (accessed October 2011).

14. Mehlisch, D. R. "Ketoprofen, Ibuprofen, and Placebo in the Treatment of Primary Dysmenorrhea: A Double-Blind Crossover Comparison." *J Clin Pharmacol* 28(12 Suppl) (Dec 1988):S29-S33. Kauppila, A., L. Rönnberg. "Naproxen Sodium in Dysmenorrhea Secondary to Endometriosis." *Obstet Gynecol* 65(3) (Mar 1985):379–383.

15. U.S. National Library of Medicine National Institutes of Health. "Endometriosis." http://www.ncbi.nlm.nih.gov/pubmedhealth/PMH0001913. (accessed October 2011).

16. Ibid.

17. Ibid.

18. Ibid.

19. Proctor, M. L., P. A. Murphy. "Herbal and Dietary Therapies for Primary and Secondary Dysmenorrhoea." *Cochrane Database Syst Rev.* 3 (2001):CD002124.

20. Parazzini, F., F. Chiaffarino, M. Surace, et al. "Selected Food Intake and Risk of Endometriosis." *Hum Reprod* 19(8) (Aug 2004):1755–1759.

21. United States Department of Agriculture. "USDA and HHS Announce New Dietary Guidelines to Help Americans Make Healthier Food Choices and Confront Obesity Epidemic." http://www.cnpp.usda.gov/Publications/DietaryGuidelines/2010/PolicyDoc/PressRelease.pdf. (accessed November 2011).

22. Endometriosis.org. "Treatments." http://www.endometriosis.org/treatments/. (accessed November 2011).

23. Shepperson Mills, D. "Nutritional Therapy Provides an Effective Method of Improving Fertility Rates and Reducing Abdominal Pain in Women with Endometriosis." *Fertil Steril* 86(3, Suppl) (Sept 2006):S270-S271.

24. Ibid.

25. Endometriosis.org. "Dietary Modification to Alleviate Endometriosis Symptoms: Interview between Nutritionist Dian Shepperson Mills and Dr. Mark Perloe." http://endometriosis.org/resources/articles/dietary-modification/. (accessed November 2011).

26. Wang, L., X. Wang, W. Wang, et al. "Stress and Dysmenorrhoea: A Population Based Prospective Study." *Occup Environ Med* 61(12) (Dec 2004): 1021–1026.

27. Akin, M., W. Price, G. Rodriguez Jr., et al. "Continuous, Low-Level, Topical Heat Wrap Therapy as Compared to Acetaminophen for Primary Dysmenorrhea." *J Reprod Med* 49(9) (Sep 2004):739–745. Akin, M. D., K. W. Weingand, D. A.

Hengehold, et al. "Continuous Low-Level Topical Heat in the Treatment of Dysmenorrhea." *Obstet Gynecol* 97(3) (Mar 2001):343–349.

28. Seifert, B., P. Wagler, S. Dartsch, et al. "[Magnesium—A New Therapeutic Alternative in Primary Dysmenorrhea]." *Zentralbl Gynakol* 111(11) (1989):755–760. Lefebvre, G., O. Pinsonneault, V. Antao, et al. "Primary Dysmenorrhea Consensus Guideline." *J Obstet Gynaecol Can* 27(12) (Dec 2005):1117–1146. Fontana-Klaiber, H. and B. Hogg. "[Therapeutic Effects of Magnesium in Dysmenorrhea]." *Schweiz Rundsch Med Prax* 79(16) (Apr 17, 1990):491–494.

29. Office of Dietary Supplements. National Institutes of Health. "Magnesium." http://ods.od.nih.gov/factsheets/magnesium. (accessed November 2011).

30. Ibid.

31. Thys-Jacobs, S., P. Starkey, D. Bernstein, et al. "Calcium Carbonate and the Premenstrual Syndrome: Effects on Premenstrual and Menstrual Symptoms. Premenstrual Syndrome Study Group." *Am J Obstet Gynecol* 179(2) (Aug 1998): 444–452.

32. Gokhale, L. B. "Curative Treatment of Primary (Spasmodic) Dysmenorrhoea." *Indian J Med Res* 103 (Apr 1996):227–231.

33. Werbach, M. R., J. Moss. *Textbook of Nutritional Medicine.* Tarzana, CA: Third Line Press, 1999.

34. Lefebvre, G., O. Pinsonneault, V. Antao, et al. "Primary Dysmenorrhea Consensus Guideline." *J Obstet Gynaecol Can* 27(12) (Dec 2005):1117–1146.

35. Werbach, M. R., J. Moss. *Textbook of Nutritional Medicine.* Tarzana, CA: Third Line Press, 1999.

36. Looker, A. C., P. R. Dallman, M. D. Carroll, et al. "Prevalence of Iron Deficiency in the United States." *JAMA* 277(12) (Mar 26, 1997): 973–976.

37. U. S. Department of Health and Human Services. National Institutes of Health. National Heart Lung and Blood Institute. "Who Is at Risk for Iron-Deficiency Anemia?" http://www.nhlbi.nih.gov/health/health-topics/topics/ida/atrisk .html. (accessed November 2011). U. S. Department of Health and Human Services. National Institutes of Health. National Heart Lung and Blood Institute. "What Are the Signs and Symptoms of Iron-Deficiency Anemia?" http:// www.nhlbi.nih.gov/health/health-topics/topics/ida/signs.html. (accessed November 2011).

38. Centers for Disease Control. "Iron deficiency—United States, 1999–2000." *MMWR* 51(40) (Oct 11, 2002):897–899. Available online: http://www.cdc.gov/ mmwr/preview/ mmwrhtml/mm5140a1.htm.

39. Ulukus, M., A. Arici. "Immunology of Endometriosis." *Minerva Ginecol* 57(3) (Jun 2005):237–248.

40. Ibid.

41. Sinaii, N., S. D. Cleary, M. L. Ballweg, et al. "High rates of Autoimmune and

Endocrine Disorders, Fibromyalgia, Chronic Fatigue Syndrome and Atopic Diseases among Women with Endometriosis: A Survey Analysis." *Hum Reprod* 17(10) (Oct 2002):2715–2724.

42. Gemmill, J. A., P. Stratton, S. D. Cleary, et al. "Cancers, Infections, and Endocrine Diseases in Women with Endometriosis." *Fertil Steril* 94(5) (Oct 2010):1627–1631.

43. Butler, E. B. E. McKnight. "Vitamin E in the Treatment of Primary Dysmenorrhoea." *Lancet* 268(6869) (Apr 1955):844–847.

44. Ziaei, S. M. Zakeri, A. Kazemnejad. "A Randomised Controlled Trial of Vitamin E in the Treatment of Primary Dysmenorrhoea." *BJOG* 112(4) (Apr 2005):466–469.

45. Santanam, N., N. Kavtaradze, C. Dominguez, et al. "Antioxidant Supplementation Reduces Total Chemokines and Inflammatory Cytokines in Women with Endometriosis." *Fertil Steril* 80(Supp 3) (Sep 2003):32–33.

46. Ibid.

47. Ibid.

48. Balch, J. F., P. A. Balch. *Prescriptions for Natural Healing.* New York, NY: Avery Publishing Group, 1990.

49. Mier-Cabrera, J., T. Aburto-Soto, S. Burrola-Méndez, et al. "Women with Endometriosis Improved Their Peripheral Antioxidant Markers after the Application of a High Antioxidant Diet." *Reprod Biol Endocrinol* 7(54) (2009). Hernández Guerrero, C. A., L. Bujalil Montenegro, J. de la Jara Díaz, et al. "[Endometriosis and Deficient Intake of Antioxidants Molecules Related to Peripheral and Peritoneal Oxidative Stress]" *Ginecol Obstet Mex* 74(1) (Jan 2006):20–28. Mier-Cabrera, J., L. Jiménez-Zamudio, E. García-Latorre, et al. "Quantitative and Qualitative Peritoneal Immune Profiles, T-Cell Apoptosis and Oxidative Stress-Associated Characteristics in Women with Minimal and Mild Endometriosis." *BJOG* 118(1) (Jan 2011):6–16.

50. Missmer, S. A., J. E. Chavarro, S. Malspeis, et al. "A Prospective Study of Dietary Fat Consumption and Endometriosis Risk." *Hum Reprod* 25(6) (Jun 2010):1528–1535.

51. Mehendale, S. S., A. S. Kilari Bams, C. S. Deshmukh, et al. "Oxidative Stress-Mediated Essential Polyunsaturated Fatty Acid Alterations in Female Infertility." *Hum Fertil (Camb)* 12(1) (Mar 2009):28–33.

52. Werbach, M. R., J. Moss. *Textbook of Nutritional Medicine.* Tarzana, CA: Third Line Press, 1999. Harel, Z., F. M. Biro, R. K. Kottenhahn, et al. "Supplementation with Omega-3 Polyunsaturated Fatty Acids in the Management of Dysmenorrhea in Adolescents." *Am J Obstet Gynecol* 174(4) (1996):1335–1338.

53. Deutch, B., E. B. Jørgensen, J. C. Hansen. "Menstrual Discomfort in Danish Women Reduced by Dietary Supplements of Omega-3 PUFA and B_{12} (Fish Oil or Seal Oil Capsules)." *Nutr Res* 20(5) (2000):621–631.

54. Holoch, K. J., B. A. Lessey. "Endometriosis and Infertility." *Clin Obstet Gynecol* 53(2) (Jun 2010):429–438.

55. Hughes, E. G., D. M. Fedorkow, J. A. Collins. "A Quantitative Overview of Controlled Trials in Endometriosis-Associated Infertility." *Fertil Steril* 59(5) (May 1993):963–970.

56. Adamson, G. D., D. J. Pasta. "Surgical Treatment of Endometriosis-Associated Infertility: Meta-Analysis Compared with Survival Analysis." *Am J Obstet Gynecol* 171(6) (Dec 1994):1488–1504.

57. Grodstein, F., M. B. Goldman, D. W. Cramer. "Infertility in Women and Moderate Alcohol Use." *Am J Public Health* 84:9 (1994): 1429–1432. Grodstein, F., M. B. Goldman, D. W. Cramer. "Endometriosis and Moderate Alcohol Use: Grodstein and Colleagues Respond." Letter. *Am J Public Health* 85(7) (Jul 1995):1021–1022.

58. Bérubé, S., S. Marcoux, R. Maheux. "Characteristics Related to the Prevalence of Minimal or Mild Endometriosis in Infertile Women. Canadian Collaborative Group on Endometriosis." *Epidemiology* 9(5) (Sep 1998):504–510. Grodstein, F., M. B. Goldman, L. Ryan, et al. "Relation of Female Infertility to Consumption of Caffeinated Beverages." *Am J Epidemiol* 137(12) (Jun 15, 1993):1353–1360.

59. Jensen, T. K., T. B. Henriksen, N. H. Hjollund, et al. "Caffeine Intake and Fecundability: A Follow-Up Study among 430 Danish Couples Planning Their First Pregnancy." *Reprod Toxicol* 12(3) (May 6, 1998):289–295.

60. Andrade, A. Z., J. K. Rodrigues, L. A. Dib, et al. "[Serum Markers of Oxidative Stress in Infertile Women with Endometriosis]." *Rev Bras Ginecol Obstet* 32(6) (Jun 2010):279–285.

61. Westphal, L. M., M. L. Polan, A. S. Trant, et al. "A Nutritional Supplement for Improving Fertility in Women: A Pilot Study." *J Reprod Med* 49(4) (Apr 2004):289–293.

62. Henmi, H., T. Endo, Y. Kitajima, et al. "Effects of Ascorbic Acid Supplementation on Serum Progesterone Levels in Patients with a Luteal Phase Defect." *Fertil Steril* 80(2) (Aug 2003):459–461.

63. Ibid.

64. Chavarro, J. E., J. W. Rich-Edwards, B. A. Rosner, et al. "Use of Multivitamins, Intake of B Vitamins and Risk of Ovulatory Infertility." *Fertil Steril* 89(3) (Mar 2008):668–676.

65. Chavarro, J. E., J. W. Rich-Edwards, B. A. Rosner, et al. "Iron Intake and Risk of Ovulatory Infertility." *Obstet Gynecol* 108(5) (Nov 2006):1145–1152.

66. Balch, J. F., P. A. Balch. *Prescriptions for Natural Healing.* New York, NY: Avery Publishing Group, 1990. Werbach, M. R., J. Moss. *Textbook of Nutritional Medicine.* Tarzana, CA: Third Line Press, 1999.

CHAPTER 9. INFERTILITY—TROUBLE GETTING, AND STAYING, PREGNANT

1. Augood, C., K. Duckitt, A. A. Templeton. "Smoking and Female Infertility: A Systematic Review and Meta-Analysis." *Hum Reprod* 13(6) (1998):1532–1539.

2. Buck, G.M., L. E. Sever, R. E. Batt, et al. "Life-Style Factors and Female Infertility." *Epidemiology* 8(4) (Jul 1997):435–441. Mueller, B. A., J. R. Daling, N. S. Weiss, et al. "Recreational Drug Use and the Risk of Primary Infertility." *Epidemiology* 1(3) (May 1990):195–200.

3. Witting, A., N. Stella. "Effects of Delta-9-tetrahydrocannabinol on Human Sperm Function." *Fertility Weekly* (Mar 13, 2006):10–11.

4. Hakim, R. B., R. H. Gray, H. Zacur. "Alcohol and Caffeine Consumption and Decreased Fertility." *Fertil Steril* 70(4) (Oct 1998):632–637.

5. Grodstein, F., M. B. Goldman, and D. W. Cramer. "Infertility in Women and Moderate Alcohol Use." *Am J Public Health* 84(9) (Sep 1994):1429–1432.

6. Jensen, T. K., N. H. Hjollund, T. B. Henriksen, et al. "Does Moderate Alcohol Consumption Affect Fertility? Follow Up Study among Couples Planning First Pregnancy." *Brit Med J* 317(7157) (Aug 22, 1998):505–510.

7. Grodstein, F., M. B. Goldman, and D. W. Cramer. "Infertility in Women and Moderate Alcohol Use." *Am J Public Health* 84(9) (Sep 1994):1429–1432.

8. Grodstein, F., M. B. Goldman, L. Ryan, et al. "Relation of Female Infertility to Consumption of Caffeinated Beverages." *Am J Epidemiol* 137(12) (Jun 15, 1993):1353–1360. Jensen, T. K., T. B. Henriksen, N. H. Hjollund, et al. "Caffeine Intake and Fecundability: A Follow-Up Study among 430 Danish Couples Planning Their First Pregnancy." *Reprod Toxicol* 12(3) (May 6, 1998):289–295. Stanton, C. K., R. H. Gray. "Effects of Caffeine Consumption on Delayed Conception." *Am J Epidemiol* 142(12) (1995):1322–1329.

9. Harvard Health Publications. Harvard Medical School. "Benefit of Drinking Green Tea: The Proof is In—Drinking Tea is Healthy, Says Harvard Women's Health Watch." September 2004. http://www.health.harvard.edu/press_releases/benefit_of_drinking_green_tea. (accessed November 2011).

10. Buck, G. M., J. E. Vena, E. F. Schisterman, et al. "Parental Consumption of Contaminated Sport Fish from Lake Ontario and Predicted Fecundability." *Epidemiology* 11(4) (Jul 2000):388–393.

11. Werbach, M. R., J. Moss. *Textbook of Nutritional Medicine.* Tarzana, CA: Third Line Press, 1999. Choy, C. M., C. W. Lam, L. T. Cheung, et al. "Infertility, Blood Mercury Concentrations and Dietary Seafood Consumption: A Case-Control Study." *BJOG* 109(10) Oct 2002):1121–1125.

12. Mehendale, S. S., A. S. Kilari Bams, C. S. Deshmukh, et al. "Oxidative Stress-Mediated Essential Polyunsaturated Fatty Acid Alterations in Female Infertility." *Hum Fertil (Camb)* 12(1) (Mar 2009):28–33.

13. Orthomolecular Medicine News Service. "Vitamin Supplements Help Protect Children from Heavy Metals, Reduce Behavioral Disorders." October 8, 2007.

http://orthomolecular.org/resources/omns/v03n07.shtml. (accessed November 2011).

14. Balch, J. F., P. A. Balch. *Prescriptions for Natural Healing*. New York, NY: Avery Publishing Group, 1990.

15. Missmer, S. A., J. E. Chavarro, S. Malspeis, et al. "A Prospective Study of Dietary Fat Consumption and Endometriosis Risk." *Hum Reprod* 25(6) (Jun 2010):1528–1535.

16. Parazzini, F., F. Chiaffarino, M. Surace, et al. "Selected Food Intake and Risk of Endometriosis." *Hum Reprod* 19(8) (Aug 2004):1755–1759.

17. Ibid.

18. Green, B. B., N. S. Weiss, J. R. Daling. "Risk of Ovulatory Infertility in Relation to Body Weight." *Fertil Steril* 50(5) (Nov 1988):721–726.

19. Ferguson, R., G. K. Holmes, W. T. Cooke. "Coeliac Disease, Fertility, and Pregnancy." *Scand J Gastroenterol* 17(1) (Jan 1982):65–68. Sher, K. S., J. F. Mayberry. "Female Fertility, Obstetric and Gynaecological History in Coeliac Disease: A Case Control Study." *Acta Paediatr Suppl* 412 (May 1996):76–77. Martinelli, P., R. Troncone, F. Paparo, et al. "Coeliac Disease and Unfavourable Outcome of Pregnancy." *Gut* 46(3) (Mar 2000):332–335. Eliakim, R., D. M. Sherer. "Celiac Disease: Fertility and Pregnancy." *Gynecol Obstet Invest* 51(1) (2001):3–7. Pellicano, R., M. Astegiano, M. Bruno, et al. "Women and Celiac Disease: Association with Unexplained Infertility." *Minerva Med* 98(3) (Jun 2007):217–219. Soni, S., S. Z. Badawy. "Celiac Disease and Its Effect on Human Reproduction: A Review." *J Reprod Med* 55(1–2) (Jan-Feb 2010):3–8.

20. Shames, R. L., K. H. Shames. *Thyroid Power: Ten Steps to Total Health*. New York, NY: HarperResource, 2001.

21. Ibid.

22. Prevention Health Books. *Prevention's Best Vitamin Cures: The Ultimate Compendium of Vitamin and Mineral Cures with More than 500 Remedies for Whatever Ails You!*. New York: Rodale; St. Martin's Paperbacks, 2000.

23. Ibid.

24. Andrade, A. Z., J. K. Rodrigues, L. A. Dib, et al. "[Serum Markers of Oxidative Stress in Infertile Women with Endometriosis]." *Rev Bras Ginecol Obstet* 32(6) (Jun 2010):279–285. Sekhon, L. H., S. Gupta, Y. Kim, et al. "Female Infertility and Antioxidants." *Curr Women's Health Rev* 6(2) (2010):84–95. Vural, P., C. Akgül, A. Yildirim, et al. "Antioxidant Defence in Recurrent Abortion." *Clin Chim Acta* 295(1–2) (May 2000):169–177. Nelen, W. L., H. J. Blom, E. A. Steegers, et al. "Hyperhomocysteinemia and Recurrent Early Pregnancy Loss: A Meta-Analysis." *Fertil Steril* 74(6) (Dec 2000):1196–1199.

25. Chavarro J. E., J. W. Rich-Edwards, B. Rosner, et al. "Use of Multivitamins, Intake of B Vitamins, and Risk of Ovulatory Infertility." *Fertil Steril* 89(3) (Mar 2008):668–676.

26. Westphal, L. M., M. L. Polan, A. S. Trant, et al. "A Nutritional Supplement for Improving Fertility in Women: A Pilot Study." *J Reprod Med* 49(4) (Apr 2004):289–293.

27. Chavarro, J. E., J. W. Rich-Edwards, B. A. Rosner, et al. "Iron Intake and Risk of Ovulatory Infertility." *Obstet Gynecol* 108(5) (Nov 2006):1145–1152.

28. Henmi, H., T. Endo, Y. Kitajima, et al. "Effects of Ascorbic Acid Supplementation on Serum Progesterone Levels in Patients with a Luteal Phase Defect." *Fertil Steril* 80(2) (Aug 2003):459–461.

29. Al-Azemi, M. K., A. E. Omu, T. Fatinikun, et al. "Factors Contributing to Gender Differences in Serum Retinol and ?-Ttocopherol in Infertile Couples." *Reprod Biomed Online* 19(4) (Oct 2009):583–590.

30. Czeizel, A. E. "Periconceptional Folic Acid Containing Multivitamin Supplementation." *Eur J Obstet Gynecol Reprod Biol* 78(2) (Jun 1998):151–161.

31. Howard, J. M., S. Davies, A. Hunnisett. "Red Cell Magnesium and Glutathione Peroxidase in Infertile Women—Effects of Oral Supplementation with Magnesium and Selenium." *Magnes Res* 7(1) (1994):49–57.

32. Balch, J. F., P. A. Balch. *Prescriptions for Natural Healing*. New York, NY: Avery Publishing Group, 1990.

33. PubMed Health. A. D. A. M. Medical Encyclopedia. "Polycystic Ovary Syndrome." http://www.ncbi.nlm.nih.gov/pubmedhealth/PMH0001408/. (accessed November 2011).

34. Mayo Clinic. "Polycystic Ovary Syndrome." http://www.mayoclinic.com/health/polycystic-ovary-syndrome/DS00423. (accessed November 2011).

35. Ibid.

36. PubMed Health. A. D. A. M. Medical Encyclopedia. "Polycystic Ovary Syndrome." http://www.ncbi.nlm.nih.gov/pubmedhealth/PMH0001408/. (accessed November 2011).

37. Lydic, M., V. Juturu. "Dietary Approaches and Alternative Therapies for Polycystic Ovary Syndrome." *Curr Nutr Food Sci* 4(4) (Nov 2008):265–281.

38. Lucidi, S., A. Thyer, C. Easton, et al. "Effect of Chromium Supplementation on Insulin Resistance and Ovarian and Menstrual Cyclicity in Women with Polycystic Ovary Syndrome." *Fertil Steril* 84(6) (Dec 2005):1755–1757.

39. Balch, J. F., P. A. Balch. *Prescriptions for Natural Healing*. New York, NY: Avery Publishing Group, 1990.

40. Lanzafame, F. M., S. La Vignera, E. Vicari, et al. "Oxidative Stress and Medical Antioxidant Treatment in Male Infertility." *Reprod Biomed Online* 19(5) (Nov 2009):638–659.

41. Ross, C., A. Morriss, M. Khairy, et al. "A Systematic Review of the Effect of Oral Antioxidants on Male Infertility." *Reprod Biomed Online* 20(6) (Jun 2010): 711–723.

42. Werbach, M. R., J. Moss. *Textbook of Nutritional Medicine.* Tarzana, CA: Third Line Press, 1999. Al-Azemi, M. K., A. E. Omu, T. Fatinikun, et al. "Factors Contributing to Gender Differences in Serum Retinol and ?-Ttocopherol in Infertile Couples." *Reprod Biomed Online* 19(4) (Oct 2009):583–590.

43, Centers for Disease Control and Prevention. "Pelvic Inflammatory Disease (PID)-CDC Fact Sheet." http://www.cdc.gov/std/pid/stdfact-pid.htm. (accessed November 2011).

44. U. S. Department of Health and Human Services. Office on Women's Health. Womenshealth.gov. "Infertility Fact Sheet." http://www.womenshealth.gov/publications/our-publications/fact-sheet/infertility.cfm#a. (accessed November 2011).

45. Sekhon, L. H., S. Gupta, Y. Kim, et al. "Female Infertility and Antioxidants." *Curr Women's Health Rev* 6(2) (2010):84–95. Bedwal, R. S., and A. Bahuguna. "Zinc, Copper and Selenium in Reproduction." *Experientia* 50(7) (Jul 15, 1994):626–640.

46. Sekhon, L. H., S. Gupta, Y. Kim, et al. "Female Infertility and Antioxidants." *Curr Women's Health Rev* 6(2) (2010):84–95.

47. Vural, P., C. Akgül, A. Yildirim, et al. "Antioxidant Defence in Recurrent Abortion." *Clin Chim Acta* 295(1–2) (May 2000):169–177.

48. Nelen, W. L., H. J. Blom, E. A. Steegers, et al. "Hyperhomocysteinemia and Recurrent Early Pregnancy Loss: A Meta-Analysis." *Fertil Steril* 74(6) (Dec 2000):1196–1199.

49. Reznikoff-Etiévant M. F., J. Zittoun, C. Vaylet, et al. "Low Vitamin B(12) Level as a Risk Factor for Very Early Recurrent Abortion." *Eur J Obstet Gynecol Reprod Biol* 104(2) (Sep 10, 2002):156–159.

CHAPTER 10. SEX DRIVE . . . WAIT . . . WHAT?

1. Brody, S. "High-dose Ascorbic Acid Increases Intercourse Frequency and Improves Mood: A Randomized Controlled Clinical Trial." *Biol Psychiatry* 52(4) (Aug 2002):371–374.

2. Ibid.

3. Ibid.

4. Coppen, A., C. Bolander-Gouaille. "Treatment of Depression: Time to Consider Folic Acid and Vitamin B_{12}." *J Psychopharmacol* 19(1) (Jan 2005):59–65.

5. Werbach, M. R., J. Moss. *Textbook of Nutritional Medicine.* Tarzana, CA: Third Line Press, 1999. Heap, L. C., T. J. Peters, S. Wessely. "Vitamin B Status in Patients with Chronic Fatigue Syndrome." *J R Soc Med* 92(4) (Apr 1999): 183–185.

6. Shipowick, C. D., C. B. Moore, C. Corbett, et al. "Vitamin D and Depressive Symptoms in Women During the Winter: A Pilot Study." *Appl Nurs Res* 22(3) (Aug 2009):221–225.

7. U. S. Department of Health and Human Services. National Institutes of Health.

National Heart Lung and Blood Institute. "Who Is at Risk for Iron-Deficiency Anemia?" http://www.nhlbi.nih.gov/health/health-topics/topics/ida/atrisk.html. (accessed November 2011).

8. U. S. Department of Health and Human Services. National Institutes of Health. National Heart Lung and Blood Institute. "What Are the Signs and Symptoms of Iron-Deficiency Anemia?" http://www.nhlbi.nih.gov/health/health-topics/topics/ida/signs.html. (accessed November 2011).

9. Verdon, F., B. Burnand, C-L Fallab Stubi, et al. "Iron Supplementation for Unexplained Fatigue in Non-Anaemic Women: Double Blind Randomised Placebo Controlled Trial." *Brit Med J* 326(7399) (May 24, 2003):1124.

CHAPTER 11. MENOPAUSE: BEFORE, DURING, AND AFTER

1. U. S. National Library of Medicine. PubMed Health. "Menopause: Perimenopause; Postmenopause." http://www.ncbi.nlm.nih.gov/pubmedhealth/PMH 0001896/. (accessed November 2011). Dean, C. *Hormone Balance: A Woman's Guide to Restoring Health and Vitality.* Avon, MA: Adams Media, 2005.

2. U. S. National Library of Medicine. PubMed Health. "Menopause: Perimenopause; Postmenopause." http://www.ncbi.nlm.nih.gov/pubmedhealth/PMH 0001896/. (accessed November 2011).

3. U.S. National Library of Medicine. National Institutes of Health. Medline Plus. "Hormone Therapy." http://www.nlm.nih.gov/medlineplus/ency/article/007111.htm. (accessed November 2011).

4. Rossouw, J. E., G. L. Anderson, R. L. Prentice, et al. "Risks and Benefits of Estrogen Plus Progestin in Healthy Postmenopausal Women: Principal Results From the Women's Health Initiative Randomized Controlled Trial." *J Amer Med Assoc* 288(3) (2002): 321–333.

5. Ibid.

6. U.S. National Library of Medicine. National Institutes of Health. Medline Plus. "Hormone Therapy." http://www.nlm.nih.gov/medlineplus/ency/article/007111.htm. (accessed November 2011).

7. Vihtamäki, T., R. Savilahti, R. Tuimala. "Why Do Postmenopausal Women Discontinue Hormone Replacement Therapy?" *Maturitas* 33(2) (Oct 1999):99–105.

8. Schuetz, F., I. J. Diel, M. Pueschel, et al. "Reduced Incidence of Distant Metastases and Lower Mortality in 1072 Patients with Breast Cancer with a History of Hormone Replacement Therapy." *Am J Obstet Gynecol* 196(4) (Apr 2007): 342.e1–9.

9. Dean, C. *Hormone Balance: A Woman's Guide to Restoring Health and Vitality.* Avon, MA: Adams Media, 2005. Balch, J. F., P. A. Balch. *Prescriptions for Natural Healing.* New York, NY: Avery Publishing Group, 1990.

10. Walker, A. F., M. C. Souza, M. F. Vickers, et al. "Magnesium Supplementation Alleviates Premenstrual Symptoms of Fluid Retention." *J Womens Health* 7(9) (Nov 1998):1157–1165.

11. Balch, J. F., P. A. Balch. *Prescriptions for Natural Healing.* New York, NY: Avery Publishing Group, 1990.

12. Thys-Jacobs, S., P. Starkey, D. Bernstein, et al. "Calcium Carbonate and the Premenstrual Syndrome: Effects on Premenstrual and Menstrual Symptoms. Premenstrual Syndrome Study Group." *Am J Obstet Gynecol* 179(2) (Aug 1998): 444–452. Thys-Jacobs, S., S. Ceccarelli, A. Bierman, et al. "Calcium Supplementation in Premenstrual Syndrome: A Randomized Crossover Trial." *J Gen Intern Med* 4(3) (May-Jun 1989):183–189.

13. Faure, E. D, P. Chantre, P. Mares. "Effects of a Standardized Soy Extract on Hot Flushes: A Multicenter, Double-Blind, Randomized, Placebo-Controlled Study." *Menopause* 9(5) (Sep-Oct 2002):329–334.

14. Upmalis, D. H., R. Lobo, L. Bradley, et al. "Vasomotor Symptom Relief by Soy Isoflavone Extract Tablets in Postmenopausal Women: A Multicenter, Double-Blind, Randomized, Placebo-Controlled Study." *Menopause* 7(4) (Jul-Aug 2000):236–242.

15. Albertazzi, P., F. Pansini, G. Bonaccorsi, et al. "The Effect of Dietary Soy Supplementation on Hot Flushes." *Obstet Gynecol* 91(1) (Jan 1998):6–11.

16. Dean, C. *Hormone Balance: A Woman's Guide to Restoring Health and Vitality.* Avon, MA: Adams Media, 2005.

17. Balch, J. F., P. A. Balch. *Prescriptions for Natural Healing.* New York, NY: Avery Publishing Group, 1990.

18. Ibid.

19. Ibid.

20. Ibid.

21. Dean, C. *Hormone Balance: A Woman's Guide to Restoring Health and Vitality.* Avon, MA: Adams Media, 2005.

22. Yildirim, B., B. Kaleli, E. Düzcan, et al. "The Effects of Postmenopausal Vitamin D Treatment on Vaginal Atrophy." *Maturitas* 49(4) (Dec 10, 2004):334–337.

23. Badalian, S. S., P. F. Rosenbaum. "Vitamin D and Pelvic Floor Disorders in Women: Results from the National Health and Nutrition Examination Survey." *Obstet Gynecol* 115(4) (Apr 2010):795–803.

24. Dallosso, H. M., C. W. McGrother, R. J. Matthews, et al. "Nutrient Composition of the Diet and the Development of Overactive Bladder: A Longitudinal Study in Women." *Neurourol Urodyn* 23(3) (2004):204–210.

25. Berghmans, L. C., H. J. Hendriks, K. Bo, et al. "Conservative Treatment of Stress Urinary Incontinence in Women: A Systematic Review of Randomized Clinical Trials." *Brit J Urol* 82(2) (Aug 1998):181–191.

26. Dean, C. *Hormone Balance: A Woman's Guide to Restoring Health and Vitality.* Avon, MA: Adams Media, 2005.

27. Balch, J. F., P. A. Balch. *Prescriptions for Natural Healing.* New York, NY: Avery Publishing Group, 1990.

28. Challem, J. *The Food Mood Solution.* Hoboken, NJ: John Wiley & Sons, 2007.

29. Zeisel, S. H. "Choline: Needed for Normal Development of Memory." *J Am Coll Nutr* 19(5 Suppl) (Oct 2000):528S-531S.

30. Ibid.

31. Balch, J. F., P. A. Balch. *Prescriptions for Natural Healing.* New York, NY: Avery Publishing Group, 1990.

32. Prevention Health Books. *Prevention's Best Vitamin Cures: The Ultimate Compendium of Vitamin and Mineral Cures with More than 500 Remedies for Whatever Ails You!.* New York: Rodale; St. Martin's Paperbacks, 2000. Darnell, L. S., H. H. Sandstead. "Iron, Zinc and Cognition of Women." *Am J Clin Nutr* 53(3) (Mar 1991):16. (Abstract).

33. Kaufman, W. *The Common Form of Joint Dysfunction.* Brattleboro, VT: E.L. Hildreth and Co., 1949. Pages 20–29 available online at: http://www.DoctorYourself.com/kaufman5.html. (accessed November 2011).

34. Balch, J. F., P. A. Balch. *Prescriptions for Natural Healing.* New York, NY: Avery Publishing Group, 1990.

35. Ibid.

36. Dean, C. *Hormone Balance: A Woman's Guide to Restoring Health and Vitality.* Avon, MA: Adams Media, 2005.

37. Ibid.

38. Lee, C. J., G. S. Lawler, G. H. Johnson. "Effects of Supplementation of the Diets with Calcium and Calcium-Rich Foods on Bone Density of Elderly Females with Osteoporosis." Am J Clin Nutr 34(5) (May 1981):819–823.

39. Dean, C. *Hormone Balance: A Woman's Guide to Restoring Health and Vitality.* Avon, MA: Adams Media, 2005.

40. American Heart Association. "Women, Heart Disease and Stroke." http://www .heart.org/HEARTORG/General/Women-Heart-Disease-and-Stroke_UCM_310572_Article.jsp#.TsWT6Va9JOw. (accessed November 2011).

CHAPTER 12. PROTECT YOURSELF FROM CANCER: REDUCING YOUR RISK OF BREAST, OVARIAN, ENDOMETRIAL, AND CERVICAL CANCERS

1. National Institutes of Health. National Cancer Institute. "Women's Cancers." http://www.cancer.gov/cancertopics/types/womenscancers. (accessed November 2011).

2. Ibid.

3. U.S. Department of Health and Human Services. National Cancer Institute.

President's Cancer Panel: 2006–2007 Annual Report. "Promoting Healthy Lifestyles: Policy, Program, and Personal Recommendations for Reducing Cancer Risk." http://deainfo.nci.nih.gov/ advisory/pcp/annualReports/pcp07rpt/pcp07 rpt.pdf. (accessed November 2011)

4. Wynder, E. L., L. A. Cohen, J. E. Muscat, et al. "Breast Cancer: Weighing the Evidence for a Promoting Role of Dietary Fat." *J Natl Cancer Inst* 89(11) (Jun 4, 1997):766–775. Binukumar, B., A. Mathew. "Dietary Fat and Risk of Breast Cancer." *World J Surg Oncol* 18(3) (Jul 18, 2005): 45. Wu, A. H., M. C. Pike, D. O. Stram. "Meta-Analysis: Dietary Fat Intake, Serum Estrogen Levels, and the Risk of Breast Cancer." *J Natl Cancer Inst* 91(6) (Mar 17, 1999):529–534. Thiébaut, A. C., V. Kipnis, S. C. Chang, et al. "Dietary Fat and Postmenopausal Invasive Breast Cancer in the National Institutes of Health-AARP Diet and Health Study Cohort." *J Natl Cancer Inst* 99(6) (Mar 21, 2007):451–462. Huncharek, M., B. Kupelnick. "Dietary Fat Intake and Risk of Epithelial Ovarian Cancer: A Meta-Analysis of 6,689 Subjects from 8 Observational Studies." *Nutr Cancer* 40(2) (2001):87–91. Shu, X. O., W. Zheng, N. Potischman, et al. "A Population-Based Case-Control Study of Dietary Factors and Endometrial Cancer in Shanghai, People's Republic of China." *Am J Epidemiol* 137(2) (1993):155–165.

5. Huncharek, M., B. Kupelnick. "Dietary Fat Intake and Risk of Epithelial Ovarian Cancer: A Meta-Analysis of 6,689 Subjects from 8 Observational Studies." *Nutr Cancer* 40(2) (2001):87–91. Shu, X. O., W. Zheng, N. Potischman, et al. "A Population-Based Case-Control Study of Dietary Factors and Endometrial Cancer in Shanghai, People's Republic of China." *Am J Epidemiol* 137(2) (1993):155–165. Cho, E., D. Spiegelman, D. J. Hunter, et al. "Premenopausal Fat Intake and Risk of Breast Cancer." *J Natl Cancer Inst* 95(14) (Jul 16, 2003):1079–1085. Cho, E., W. Y. Chen, D. J. Hunter, et al. "Red Meat Intake and Risk of Breast Cancer among Premenopausal Women." *Arch Intern Med* 166(20) (Nov 13, 2006):2253–2259. Linos, E., W. C. Willett, E. Cho, et al. "Red Meat Consumption during Adolescence among Premenopausal Women and Risk of Breast Cancer." *Cancer Epidemiol Biomarkers Prev* 17(8) (2008): 2146–2151. Kolahdooz, F., J. C. van der Pols, C. J. Bain, et al. "Meat, Fish, and Ovarian Cancer Risk: Results from 2 Australian Case-Control Studies, a Systematic Review, and Meta-Analysis." *Am J Clin Nutr* 91(6) (Jun 2010):1752–1763.

6. Willett, W. C., M. J. Stampfer, G. A. Colditz, et al. "Relation of Meat, Fat, and Fiber Intake to the Risk of Colon Cancer in a Prospective Study among Women." *N Engl J Med* 323(24) (Dec 13, 1990):1664–1672.

7. Putnam, J., J. Allshouse, L. S. Kantor. "U.S. per Capita Food Supply Trends: More Calories, Refined Carbohydrates, and Fats." *FoodReview* 25(3) (2002):2–15. http://ers.usda.gov/publications/FoodReview/DEC2002/frvol25i3a .pdf (accessed November 2011).

8. American Cancer Society. "Breast Cancer: Causes, Risk Factors, and Prevention Topics." http://www.cancer.org/Cancer/BreastCancer/DetailedGuide/breast-cancer-risk-factors. (accessed November 2011).

9. Willett, W. C., M. J. Stampfer, G. A. Colditz, et al. "Moderate Alcohol Con-

sumption and the Risk of Breast Cancer." *N Engl J Med* 316(19) (May 7, 1987):1174–1180. Smith-Warner, S. A., D. Spiegelman, S. S. Yaun, et al. "Alcohol and Breast Cancer in Women: A Pooled Analysis of Cohort Studies." *JAMA* 279:7 (1998): 535–540. Horn-Ross, P. L., A. J. Canchola, D. W. West, et al. "Patterns of Alcohol Consumption and Breast Cancer Risk in the California Teachers Study Cohort." *Cancer Epidem Biomar* 13(3) (Mar 2004):405–411. Kuper, H. L. Titus-Ernstoff, B. L. Harlow, et al. "Population Based Study of Coffee, Alcohol and Tobacco Use and Risk of Ovarian Cancer." *Int J Cancer* 88(2) (Oct 15, 2000):313–318. Modugno, F., R. B. Ness, G. O. Allen. "Alcohol Consumption and the Risk of Mucinous and Nonmucinous Epithelial Ovarian Cancer." *Obstet Gynecol* 102(6) (Dec 2003):1336–1343. Longnecker, M. P., J. A. Berlin, M. J. Orza, et al. "A Meta-Analysis of Alcohol Consumption in Relation to Risk of Breast Cancer." *JAMA* 260(5) (1988):652–656.

10. Jordan, S. J., D. C. Whiteman, D, M. Purdie, et al. "Does Smoking Increase Risk of Ovarian Cancer? A Systematic Review." *Gynecol Oncol* 103(3) (Dec 2006):1122–1129.

11. Ibid.

12. International Collaboration of Epidemiological Studies of Cervical Cancer, P. Appleby, A. Berrington de González, et al. "Carcinoma of the Cervix and Tobacco Smoking: Collaborative Reanalysis of Individual Data on 13,541 Women with Carcinoma of the Cervix and 23,017 Women without Carcinoma of the Cervix from 23 Epidemiological Studies." *Int J Cancer* 118(6) (Mar 15, 2006): 1481–1495.

13. Baumgartner, K. B., T. J. Schlierf, D. Yang, et al. "N-Acetyltransferase 2 Genotype Modification of Active Cigarette Smoking on Breast Cancer Risk among Hispanic and Non-Hispanic White Women." *Toxicol Sci* 112(1) (2009):211–220.

14. Egan, K. M., M. J. Stampfer, D Hunter, et al. "Active and Passive Smoking in Breast Cancer: Prospective Results from the Nurses' Health Study." *Epidemiology* 13(2) (Mar 2002):138–145.

15. Schlesselman, J. J. "Net Effect of Oral Contraceptive Use on the Risk of Cancer in Women in the United States." *Obstet Gynecol* 85(5 Pt 1)(May 1995): 793–801.

16. Augustin, L. S., S. Gallus, C. Bosetti, et al. "Glycemic Index and Glycemic Load in Endometrial Cancer." *Int J Cancer* 105(3) (Jun 20, 2003):404–407. Augustin, L. S., J. Polesel, C. Bosetti, et al. "Dietary Glycemic Index, Glycemic Load and Ovarian Cancer Risk: A Case-Control Study in Italy." *Ann Oncol* 14(1) (Jan 2003):78–84. Augustin, L. S., L. Dal Maso, C. La Vecchia, et al. "Dietary Glycemic Index and Glycemic Load, and Breast Cancer Risk: A Case-Control Study." *Ann Oncol* 12(11) (Nov 2001):1533–1538.

17. United States Department of Agriculture. Center for Nutrition Policy and Promotion. "Report of the Dietary Guidelines Advisory Committee on the Dietary Guidelines for Americans, 2010. Part B. Section 2: The Total Diet: Combining Nutrients, Consuming Food." http://www.cnpp.usda.gov/Publications/Dietary Guidelines/2010/DGAC/Report/B-2-TotalDiet.pdf. (accessed November 2011).

18. Department of Health and Human Services. Centers for Disease Control. "How Many Fruits and Vegetables Do You Need?" http://www.fruitsandveggies-matter.gov/downloads/ General_Audience_Brochure.pdf. (accessed November 2011).

19. Centers for Disease Control. CDC Online Newsroom. "Majority of Americans Not Meeting Recommendations for Fruit and Vegetable Consumption." Press Release, September 29, 2009. http://www.cdc.gov/media/pressrel/2009/r090929.htm. (accessed November 2011).

20. Casagrande, S. S., Y. Wang, C. Anderson, et al. "Have Americans Increased Their Fruit and Vegetable Intake? The Trends between 1988 and 2002." *Am J Prev Med* 32(4) (Apr 2007):257–263. Available online: http://www.fruitsandveg-giesmorematters.org/wp-content/uploads/UserFiles/File/pdf/press/AJPM_32-4_Casagrande_with%20embargo.pdf. (accessed November 2011).

21. Balch, J. F., P. A. Balch. *Prescriptions for Natural Healing.* New York, NY: Avery Publishing Group, 1990.

22. U. S. Department of Agriculture. "USDA and HHS Announce New Dietary Guidelines to Help Americans Make Healthier Food Choices and Confront Obesity Epidemic." http://www.cnpp.usda.gov/Publications/DietaryGuidelines/2010/PolicyDoc/PressRelease.pdf. (accessed November 2011).

23. Gandini, S., H. Merzenich, C. Robertson, et al. "Meta-Analysis of Studies on Breast Cancer Risk and Diet: The Role of Fruit and Vegetable Consumption and the Intake of Associated Micronutrients." *Eur J Cancer* 36(5) (Mar 2000):636–646. Riboli, E., T. Norat. "Epidemiologic Evidence of the Protective Effect of Fruit and Vegetables on Cancer Risk." *Am J Clin Nutr* 78(3 Suppl) (Sep 2003):559S-569S. United States Department of Agriculture. Center for Nutrition Policy and Promotion. "Report of the Dietary Guidelines Advisory Committee on the Dietary Guidelines for Americans, 2010. Part D. Section 5: Carbohydrates." Table D4.2. http://www.cnpp.usda.gov/Publications/DietaryGuidelines/2010/DGAC/Report/D-5-Carbohydrates.pdf. (accessed November 2011). McCann, S. E, J. L. Freudenheim, J. R. Marshall, et al. "Risk of Human Ovarian Cancer is Related to Dietary Intake of Selected Nutrients, Phytochemicals and Food Groups." *J Nutr* 133(6) (Jun 2003):1937–1942.

24. Liu, S., J. E. Manson, I. M. Lee, et al. "Fruit and Vegetable Intake and Risk of Cardiovascular Disease: The Women's Health Study." *Am J Clin Nutr* 72(4) (Oct 2000):922–928. Hung, H. C., K. J. Joshipura, R. Jiang, et al. "Fruit and Vegetable Intake and Risk of Major Chronic Disease." *J Natl Cancer Inst* 96(21) (2004):1577–1584.

25. Block, G., B. Patterson, A. Subar. "Fruit, Vegetables, and Cancer Prevention: A Review of the Epidemiological Evidence." *Nutr Cancer* 18(1) (1992):1–29.

26. Blanchard, C. M., K. S. Courneya, K. Stein. "Cancer Survivors' Adherence to Lifestyle Behavior Recommendations and Associations with Health-Related Quality of Life: Results from the American Cancer Society's SCS-II." *J Clin Oncol* 26(13) (May 1, 2008): 2198–2204.

27. Reed, J., E. Frazão, R. Itskowitz. United States Department of Agriculture. Economic Research Service. "How Much Do Americans Pay for Fruits and Vegetables?" Agriculture Information Bulletin, October 2004. http://www.ers.usda .gov/publications/aib792/aib792–4/aib792–4.pdf. (accessed November 2011).

28. Ibid.

29. United States Department of Agriculture. Economic Research Service. "Access to Affordable and Nutritious Food: Measuring and Understanding Food Deserts and Their Consequences." Report to Congress, June 2009. http://www.ers.usda .gov/Publications/ AP/AP036/AP036.pdf. (accessed November 2011).

30. Ibid.

31. Sharma, A. K., P. Mohan, B. B. Nayak. "Probiotics: Making a Comeback." *Indian J Pharmacol* 37(6) (2005): 358–365. Van't Veer P., E. M. van Leer, A. Rietdijk, et al. "Combination of Dietary Factors in Relation to Breast-Cancer Occurrence." *Int J Cancer* 47(5) (Mar 12, 1991):649–653.

32. Kumar, M., A. Kumar, R. Nagpal, et al. "Cancer-Preventing Attributes of Probiotics: An Update." *Int J Food Sci Nutr* 61(5) (Aug 2010):473–496.

33. McCann, S. E, J. L. Freudenheim, J. R. Marshall, et al. "Risk of Human Ovarian Cancer is Related to Dietary Intake of Selected Nutrients, Phytochemicals and Food Groups." *J Nutr* 133(6) (Jun 2003):1937–1942. Van't Veer P., E. M. van Leer, A. Rietdijk, et al. "Combination of Dietary Factors in Relation to Breast-Cancer Occurrence." *Int J Cancer* 47(5) (Mar 12, 1991):649–653. Van't Veer P., C. M. Kolb, P. Verhoef, et al. "Dietary Fiber, Beta-Carotene and Breast Cancer: Results from a Case-Control Study." *Int J Cancer* 45(5) (May 15, 1990):825–828. Goodman, M. T., L. R. Wilkens, J. H. Hankin, et al. "Association of Soy and Fiber Consumption with the Risk of Endometrial Cancer." *Am J Epidemiol* 146(4) (1997):294–306.

34. McTiernan, A. C. Kooperberg, E. White, et al. "Recreational Physical activity and the Risk of Breast Cancer in Postmenopausal Women: The Women's Health Initiative Cohort Study." *JAMA* 290(10) (Sep 10, 2003):1331–1336. Maruti, S. S., W. C. Willett, D. Feskanich, et al. "A Prospective Study of Age-Specific Physical Activity and Premenopausal Breast Cancer." *J Natl Cancer Inst* 100(10) (2008):728–737. Thune, I., T. Brenn, E. Lund, et al. "Physical Activity and the Risk of Breast Cancer." *N Engl J Med* 336(18) (May 1, 1997): 1269–1275. Terry, P., J. A. Baron, E. Weiderpass, et al. "Lifestyle and Endometrial Cancer Risk: A Cohort Study from the Swedish Twin Registry." *Int J Cancer* 82(1) (Jul 2, 1999):38–42. Matthews, C. E., W. H. Wu, W. Zheng, et al. "Physical Activity and Risk of Endometrial Cancer: A Report from the Shanghai Endometrial Cancer Study." *Cancer Epidemiol Biomarkers Prev* 14(4) (Apr 2005):779–785. Cottreau, C. M., R. B. Ness, A. M. Kriska. "Physical Activity and Reduced Risk of Ovarian Cancer." *Obstet Gynecol* 96(4) (Oct 2000): 609–614. Dorn, J., J. Brasure, J. Freudenheim, et al. "Lifetime Physical Activity and Breast Cancer Risk in Pre- and Postmenopausal Women." *Med Sci Sports Exerc* 35(2) (Feb 2003):278–285.

35. Terry, P., J. A. Baron, E. Weiderpass, et al. "Lifestyle and Endometrial Cancer Risk: A Cohort Study from the Swedish Twin Registry." *Int J Cancer* 82(1) (Jul 2, 1999):38–42. Huang, Z., S. E. Hankinson, G. A. Colditz, et al. "Dual Effects of Weight and Weight Gain on Breast Cancer Risk." *JAMA* 278(17) (Nov 5, 1997):1407–1411. Eliassen, A. H., G. A. Colditz, B. Rosner, et al. "Adult Weight Change and Risk of Postmenopausal Breast Cancer." *JAMA* 296(2) (2006):193–201. Ballard-Barbash, R., C. A. Swanson. "Body Weight: Estimation of Risk for Breast and Endometrial Cancers." *Am J Clin Nutr* 63(3 Suppl) (1996):437S–441S. Olson, S. H., M. Trevisan, J. R. Marshall, et al. "Body Mass Index, Weight Gain, and Risk of Endometrial Cancer." *Nutr Cancer* 23(2) (1995):141–149. Lahmann, P. H., A. E. Cust, C. M. Friedenreich, et al. "Anthropometric Measures and Epithelial Ovarian Cancer Risk in the European Prospective Investigation into Cancer and Nutrition." *Int J Cancer* 126(10) (May 15, 2010):2404–2415.

36. Willett , W. C, B. MacMahon. "Diet and Cancer—An Overview." *N Engl J Med* 310(10) (Mar 15, 1984):697–703.

37. Goodman, M. T., L. R. Wilkens, J. H. Hankin, et al. "Association of Soy and Fiber Consumption with the Risk of Endometrial Cancer." *Am J Epidemiol* 146(4) (1997):294–306. Yeh, M., K. B. Moysich, V. Jayaprakash, et al. "Higher Intakes of Vegetables and Vegetable-Related Nutrients are Associated with Lower Endometrial Cancer Risks." *J Nutr* 139(2) (Feb 2009):317–322.

38. Negri, E., C. Vecchia, S. Franceschi, et al. "Intake of Selected Micronutrients and the Risk of Breast Cancer." *Int J Cancer* 65(2) (Jan 17, 1996):140–144. Verreault, R., J. Chu, M. Mandelson, et al. "A Case-Control Study of Diet and Invasive Cervical Cancer." *Int J Cancer* 43(6) (Jun 15, 1989):1050–1054.

39. ScienceDaily. "Vitamin A Pushes Breast Cancer To Form Blood Vessel Cells." ScienceDaily. July 15, 2008. http://www.sciencedaily.com/releases/2008/07/080715204719 .htm. (accessed November 2011).

40. Linus Pauling Institute. Micronutrient Information Center. "Vitamin A." http://lpi.oregonstate.edu/infocenter/vitamins/vitaminA/. (accessed November 2011).

41. Kim, K. N., J. E. Pie, J. H. Park, et al. "Retinoic Acid and Ascorbic Acid Act Synergistically in Inhibiting Human Breast Cancer Cell Proliferation." *J Nutr Biochem* 17(7) (Jul 16, 2006):454–462.

42. Michels, K. B., L. Holmberg, L. Bergkvist, et al. "Dietary Antioxidant Vitamins, Retinol, and Breast Cancer Incidence in a Cohort of Swedish Women." *Int J Cancer* 91(4) (Feb 15, 2001):563–567. Zhang, S., D. J. Hunter, M. R. Forman, et al. "Dietary Carotenoids and Vitamins A, C, and E and Risk of Breast Cancer." *J Natl Cancer Inst* 91(6) (Mar 17, 1999):547–556. Hickey, S., A. W. Saul. *Vitamin C: The Real Story.* Laguna Beach, CA: Basic Health Publications, 2008.

43. Pauling, L. *How to Live Longer and Feel Better.* Corvallis, OR: Oregon State University Press, 2006.

44. Hickey, S., H. Roberts. Orthomolecular Medicine News Service. "Vitamin C

Does Not Cause Kidney Stones." July 5, 2005. http://orthomolecular.org/resources/omns/v01n07 .shtml. (accessed November 2011).

45. Goh, Y. I., E. Bollano, T. R. Einarson, et al. "Prenatal Multivitamin Supplementation and Rates of Pediatric Cancers: A Meta-Analysis." *Clin Pharmacol Ther* 81(5) (May 2007):685–691.

46. Mursu, J., K. Robien, L. J. Harnack, et al. "Dietary Supplements and Mortality Rate in Older Women. The Iowa Women's Health Study." *Arch Intern Med* 171(18) (Oct 10, 2011):1625–1633.

47. Garland, C. F., E. D. Gorham, S. B. Mohr, et al. "Vitamin D and Prevention of Breast Cancer: Pooled Analysis." *J Steroid Biochem Mol Biol* 10(3–5) (2007):708–711.

48. Saul, A. W. "Interview with Michael Holick, M.D." DoctorYourself.Com, http://www.DoctorYourself.com/holick.html. (accessed November 2011).

49. Garland, C. F., S. B. Mohr, E. D. Gorham, et al. "Role of Ultraviolet B Irradiance and Vitamin D in Prevention of Ovarian Cancer." *Am J Prev Med* 31(6) (Dec 2006):512–514.

50. Salazar-Martinez E., E. C. Lazcano-Ponce, G. Gonzalez Lira-Lira, et al. "Nutritional Determinants of Epithelial Ovarian Cancer Risk: A Case-Control Study in Mexico." *Oncology* 63(2) (2002):151–157.

51. Thys-Jacobs, S., D. Donovan, A. Papadopoulos, et al. "Vitamin D and Calcium Dysregulation in the Polycystic Ovarian Syndrome." *Steroids* 64(6) (Jun 1999):430–435.

52. Lappe, J. M., D. Travers-Gustafson, K. M. Davies, et al. "Vitamin D and Calcium Supplementation Reduces Cancer Risk: Results of a Randomized Trial. *Am J Clin Nutr* (Jun 2007) 85(6):1586–1591.

53. Negri, E., C. Vecchia, S. Franceschi, et al. "Intake of Selected Micronutrients and the Risk of Breast Cancer." *Int J Cancer* 65(2) (Jan 17, 1996):140–144. Verreault, R., J. Chu, M. Mandelson, et al. "A Case-Control Study of Diet and Invasive Cervical Cancer." *Int J Cancer* 43(6) (Jun 15, 1989):1050–1054.

54. Yeh, M., K. B. Moysich, V. Jayaprakash, et al. "Higher Intakes of Vegetables and Vegetable-Related Nutrients are Associated with Lower Endometrial Cancer Risks." *J Nutr* 139(2) (Feb 2009):317–322.

55. Mahabir, S., K. Schendel, Y. Q. Dong et al. "Dietary Alpha-, Beta-, Gamma- and Delta-Tocopherols in Lung cancer Risk." *Int J Cancer* 123(5) (Sep 1, 2008):1173–1180.

56. American Cancer Society. "Lung Cancer (Non-Small Cell)" http://www.cancer.org/Cancer/LungCancer-Non-SmallCell/DetailedGuide/non-small-cell-lung-cancer-key-statistics. (accessed November 2011).

57. Mahabir, S., K. Schendel, Y. Q. Dong et al. "Dietary Alpha-, Beta-, Gamma- and Delta-Tocopherols in Lung cancer Risk." *Int J Cancer* 123(5) (Sep 1, 2008):1173–1180.

58. Saul, A. W. *Doctor Yourself: Natural Healing That Works.* Laguna Beach, CA: Basic Health Publications, 2003.

59. Le Marchand, L., T. Donlon, J. H. Hankin, et al. "B-Vitamin Intake, Metabolic Genes, and Colorectal Cancer Risk (United States)." *Cancer Cause Control* 13(3) (Apr 2002):239–248. Theodoratou, E., S. M. Farrington, A. Tenesa, et al. "Dietary Vitamin B_6 Intake and the Risk of Colorectal Cancer." *Cancer Epidemiol Biomarkers Prev* 17(1) (Jan 2008):171–82.

60. Yeh, M., K. B. Moysich, V. Jayaprakash, et al. "Higher Intakes of Vegetables and Vegetable-Related Nutrients are Associated with Lower Endometrial Cancer Risks." *J Nutr* 139(2) (Feb 2009):317–322.

61. Zhang, S. M., W. C. Willett, J. Selhub, et al. "Plasma Folate, Vitamin B6, Vitamin B12, Homocysteine, and Risk of Breast Cancer." *J Natl Cancer Inst* 95(5) (Mar 5, 2003):373–380. Lajous, M., E. Lazcano-Ponce, M. Hernandez-Avila, et al. "Folate, Vitamin B_6, and Vitamin B_{12} Intake and the Risk of Breast Cancer among Mexican Women." *Cancer Epidem Biomar* 15(3) (Mar 2006):443–448. Ericson, U., E. Sonestedt, B. Gullberg, et al. "High Folate Intake is Associated with Lower Breast Cancer Incidence in Postmenopausal Women in the Malmö Diet and Cancer Cohort." *Am J Clin Nutr* 86(2) (Aug 2007):434–443. Shrubsole, M. J., F. Jin, Q. Dai, et al. "Dietary Folate Intake and Breast Cancer Risk: Results from the Shanghai Breast Cancer Study." *Cancer Res* 61(19) (Oct 1, 2001):7136–7141.

62. Zhang, S., D. J. Hunter, S. E. Hankinson, et al. "A Prospective Study of Folate Intake and the Risk of Breast Cancer." *JAMA* 281(17) (May 5, 1999):1632–1637.

63. Fox News. Associated Press. "High Doses of Folic Acid May Increase Colon Cancer Risk." June 2007. http://www.foxnews.com/story/0,2933,278237,00.html. (accessed November 2011).

64. Stolzenberg-Solomon, R. Z., S. C. Chang, M. F. Leitzmann, et al. "Folate Intake, Alcohol Use, and Postmenopausal Breast Cancer Risk in the Prostate, Lung, Colorectal, and Ovarian Cancer Screening Trial." *Am J Clin Nutr* 83(4) (Apr 2006):895–904. Cole, B. F., J. A. Baron, R. S. Sandler, et al. "Folic Acid for the Prevention of Colorectal Adenomas: A Randomized Clinical Trial." *JAMA* 297(21) (2007):2351–2359.

65. Giovannucci, E., M. J. Stampfer, G. A. Colditz, et al. "Multivitamin Use, Folate, and Colon Cancer in Women in the Nurses' Health Study." *Ann Intern Med* 129(7) (Oct 1, 1998):517–524.

66. Hathcock, J. N. "Vitamins and Minerals: Efficacy and Safety." *Am J Clin Nutr* 66(2) (1997):427–37.

67. Negri, E., C. Vecchia, S. Franceschi, et al. "Intake of Selected Micronutrients and the Risk of Breast Cancer." *Int J Cancer* 65(2) (Jan 17, 1996):140–144.

68. Cho, E., S. A. Smith-Warner, D. Spiegelman, et al. "Dairy Foods, Calcium, and Colorectal Cancer: A Pooled Analysis of 10 Cohort Studies." *J Natl Cancer Inst* 96(13) (Nov 17. 2004):1015–1022.

69. Lappe, J. M., D. Travers-Gustafson, K. M. Davies, et al. "Vitamin D and Cal-

cium Supplementation Reduces Cancer Risk: Results of a Randomized Trial. *Am J Clin Nutr* (Jun 2007) 85(6):1586–1591.

70. Hathcock, J. N. "Vitamins and Minerals: Efficacy and Safety." *Am J Clin Nutr* 66(2) (1997):427–37.

71. Foster, H. D. "Selenium and Cancer: A Geographical Perspective." *J Orthomol Med* 13(1) (1998):173–175.

72. McConnell, K. P., R. M. Jager, K. I. Bland, et al. "The Relationship of Dietary Selenium and Breast Cancer." *J Surg Oncol* 15(1) (1980):67–70.

73. Cunzhi, H., J. Jiexian, Z. Xianwen, et al. "Serum and Tissue Levels of Six Trace Elements and Copper/Zinc Ratio in Patients with Cervical Cancer and Uterine Myoma." *Biol Trace Elem Res* 94(2) (Aug 2003):113–122.

74. National Institute of Health. Office of Dietary Supplements. "Dietary Supplement Fact Sheet: Selenium." http://ods.od.nih.gov/factsheets/selenium.asp. (accessed November 2011).

75. Balch, J. F., P. A. Balch. *Prescriptions for Natural Healing.* New York, NY: Avery Publishing Group, 1990.

76. Ho, E. "Zinc Deficiency, DNA Damage and Cancer Risk." *J Nutr Biochem* 15(10) (Oct 2004):572–578.

77. Gago-Dominguez, M., J. M. Yuan, C. L. Sun et al. "Opposing Effects of Dietary n-3 and n-6 Fatty Acids on Mammary Carcinogenesis: The Singapore Chinese Health Study." *Br J Cancer* 89(9) (Nov 3, 2003):1686–1692.

78. U. S. National Library of Medicine. PubMed Health. "Cervical Dysplasia." A.D.A.M. Medical Encyclopedia. http://www.ncbi.nlm.nih.gov/pubmedhealth/PMH0002461/. (accessed November 2011).

79. Liu, T. S. J. Soong, N. P. Wilson, et al. "A Case Control Study of Nutritional Factors and Cervical Dysplasia." *Cancer Epidemiol Biomarkers Prev* 2(6) (Nov-Dec 1993):525–530. Butterworth, C. E. Jr., K. D. Hatch, M. Macaluso, et al. "Folate Deficiency and Cervical Dysplasia." *JAMA* 267(4) (Jan 22–29, 1992):528–533. VanEenwyk, J., F. G. Davis, N. Colman. "Folate, Vitamin C, and Cervical Intraepithelial Neoplasia." *Cancer Epidem Biomar* 1(2) (1992):119–124. Sedjo, R. L., D. J. Roe, M. Abrahamsen, et al. "Vitamin A, Carotenoids, and Risk of Persistent Oncogenic Human Papillomavirus Infection." *Cancer Epidem Biomar* 11(9) (Sep 2002):876–884. Kwa?niewska, A., A.Tukendorf, M. Semczuk. [Frequency of HPV Infection and the Level of Ascorbic Acid in Serum of Women with Cervix Dysplasia]. *Med Dosw Mikrobiol* 48(3–4) (1996):183–188. Siegel, E. M., N. E. Craft, E. Duarte-Franco, et al. "Associations between Serum Carotenoids and Tocopherols and Type-Specific HPV Persistence: The Ludwig-McGill Cohort Study." *Int J Cancer* 120(3) (Feb 1, 2007):672–680.

80. Centers for Disease Control and Prevention (CDC). "Sexually Transmitted Diseases (STDs). Genital HPV Infection—Fact Sheet." http://www.cdc.gov/std/hpv/stdfact-hpv.htm. (accessed November 2011)

81. *Foodmatters* [DVD]. Permacology Productions, 2008.

INDEX

ABOUT THE AUTHOR

Helen Saul Case graduated *magna cum laude* from Colgate University and earned a master's degree in education from the State University of New York. She taught English for nine years, is a certified administrator, and worked as English department chair for four years. She currently lives with her husband and daughter in Western NY.

Mrs. Case has published in the *Journal of Orthomolecular Medicine*. She is the daughter of Andrew W. Saul, star of the movie *Foodmatters* and author of many popular books including *Doctor Yourself: Natural Healing that Works* and *Fire Your Doctor! How to be Independently Healthy*. Her antics as a child are featured at his well-known natural healing website www.DoctorYourself.com.

CPSIA information can be obtained
at www.ICGtesting.com
Printed in the USA
BVHW04*1423080818
523918BV00013B/198/P

9 781681 628325